Praise for

UNBLOCKED

"Clear and compelling, this book's systematic approach will help you find the obstacles that have been holding you back and release them. As your wise and compassionate guides, Margaret and David will take you on a transformational journey to your full potential. The adventure beckons!"

— **Dawson Church**, award-winning author of *Bliss Brain: The Neuroscience of Remodeling Your Brain for Resilience, Creativity, and Joy* (from the Foreword)

"A book for the "unfulfilled super achievers" trying to understand why they can't let themselves thrive and FEEL good—like they've finally arrived. If you want to stop torturing yourself, this is the book for you."

— **Jeff Walker**, *New York Times* best-selling author of *Launch*

"If you're anything like me, you devour self help books like they're going out of style. If you feel like you've tried everything when it comes to personal growth—and nothing seems to make a real difference—*Unblocked* will reveal the missing piece that has kept you from *living* what you've learned. More importantly, it will lead you directly down the path of deep, lasting change."

— **Nick Ortner**, *New York Times* best-selling author of *The Tapping Solution*

"In my years of working with leaders and entrepreneurs, I've learned that even the most successful among us are waging a silent battle with self-doubt . . . always trying to prove ourselves and secretly questioning our own worth. Margaret's approach allows us to free this stagnant energy and transform it into the unshakable confidence we need to live our best life."

— **Sage Lavine**, best-selling author of *Women Rocking Business*

"We all deeply desire to live in our power and to own our true worth, yet most of us go through life feeling like we're not enough. We try to fill the void with self-sabotaging behaviors like perfectionism, control, and over-work. The brilliance of *Unblocked* is that it goes beyond the surface and gives you foolproof tools to break the bonds that are holding you back so you can not only fill that empty space inside but you can make the contribution you were born to make in the world."

— **Debra Poneman**, best-selling author and founder of Yes to Success Seminars

"*Unblocked* is a no-nonsense approach for people who want to release deep emotional blocks that prevent them from living an exceptional life. Margaret and David's unique method focuses on the developmental issues associated with the lower chakras that hollow out the energy a person has to meet life's challenges. The book is methodical, thorough, and thought provoking, and includes very powerful visualizations.
While the book is very easy to read, it is not meant for people who are compromised or emotionally faint of heart. *Unblocked* is for people who are willing and able to deal with potentially strong emotional reactions on their journey to improve themselves. A person who dives into the ideas of the book and does the visualizations offered should be largely rewarded. Finally, even though the book is geared to the public, coaches and mental health professionals will find a rich treasure chest of ideas for helping others."

— **Robert Schwarz, PsyD, DCEP,** executive director, Association for Comprehensive Energy Psychology, author of *Tools for Transforming Trauma*

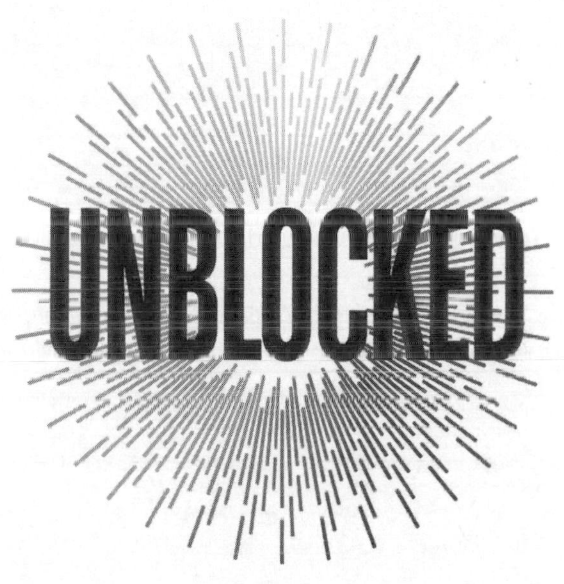
UNBLOCKED

Also by Margaret Lynch Raniere

Tapping into Wealth: How Emotional Freedom Techniques (EFT) Can Help You Clear the Path to Making More Money

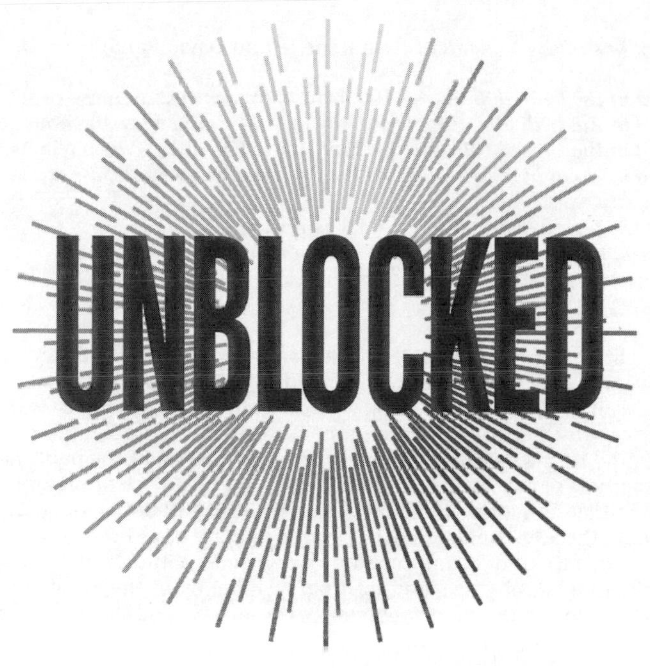

A REVOLUTIONARY APPROACH TO
Tapping into Your Chakra Empowerment Energy
to Reclaim Your Passion, Joy, and Confidence

MARGARET LYNCH RANIERE
AND DAVID RANIERE, Ph.D.

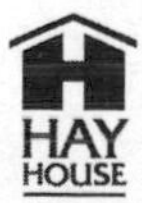

HAY HOUSE, INC.
Carlsbad, California • New York City
London • Sydney • New Delhi

Copyright © 2021 by Margaret Lynch Raniere and David Raniere, Ph.D.

Published in the United States by: Hay House, Inc.: www.hayhouse.com®
Published in Australia by: Hay House Australia Pty. Ltd.: www.hayhouse.com.au
Published in the United Kingdom by: Hay House UK, Ltd.: www.hayhouse.co.uk
Published in India by: Hay House Publishers India: www.hayhouse.co.in

Project editor: Melody Guy • *Indexer:* J S Editorial, LLC
Cover design: Barbara LeVan Fisher • *Interior design:* Nick C. Welch
Interior photos/illustrations: Courtesy of the authors

All rights reserved. No part of this book may be reproduced by any mechanical, photographic, or electronic process, or in the form of a phonographic recording; nor may it be stored in a retrieval system, transmitted, or otherwise be copied for public or private use—other than for "fair use" as brief quotations embodied in articles and reviews—without prior written permission of the publisher.

The authors of this book do not dispense medical advice or prescribe the use of any technique as a form of treatment for physical, emotional, or medical problems without the advice of a physician, either directly or indirectly. The intent of the authors is only to offer information of a general nature to help you in your quest for emotional, physical, and spiritual well-being. In the event you use any of the information in this book for yourself, the authors and the publisher assume no responsibility for your actions.

Library of Congress has cataloged the earlier edition as follows:

Names: Raniere, Margaret Lynch, author. | Raniere, David, author.
Title: Unblocked : a revolutionary approach to tapping into your chakra empowerment energy to reclaim your passion, joy, and confidence / Margaret Lynch Raniere and David Raniere, Ph.D.
Description: 1st edition. | Carlsbad, California : Hay House, Inc., 2021. | Identifiers: LCCN 2021000082 | ISBN 9781401961442 (hardback) | ISBN 9781401961459 (ebook)
Subjects: LCSH: Chakras. | Energy medicine. | Healing. | Self-actualization (Psychology)
Classification: LCC BF1442.C53 R36 2021 | DDC 131--dc23
LC record available at https://lccn.loc.gov/2021000082

Tradepaper ISBN: 978-1-4019-6545-7
E-book ISBN: 978-1-4019-6145-9
Audiobook ISBN: 978-1-4019-6146-6

10 9 8 7 6 5 4 3 2 1
1st edition, April 2021
2nd edition, April 2022

Printed in the United States of America

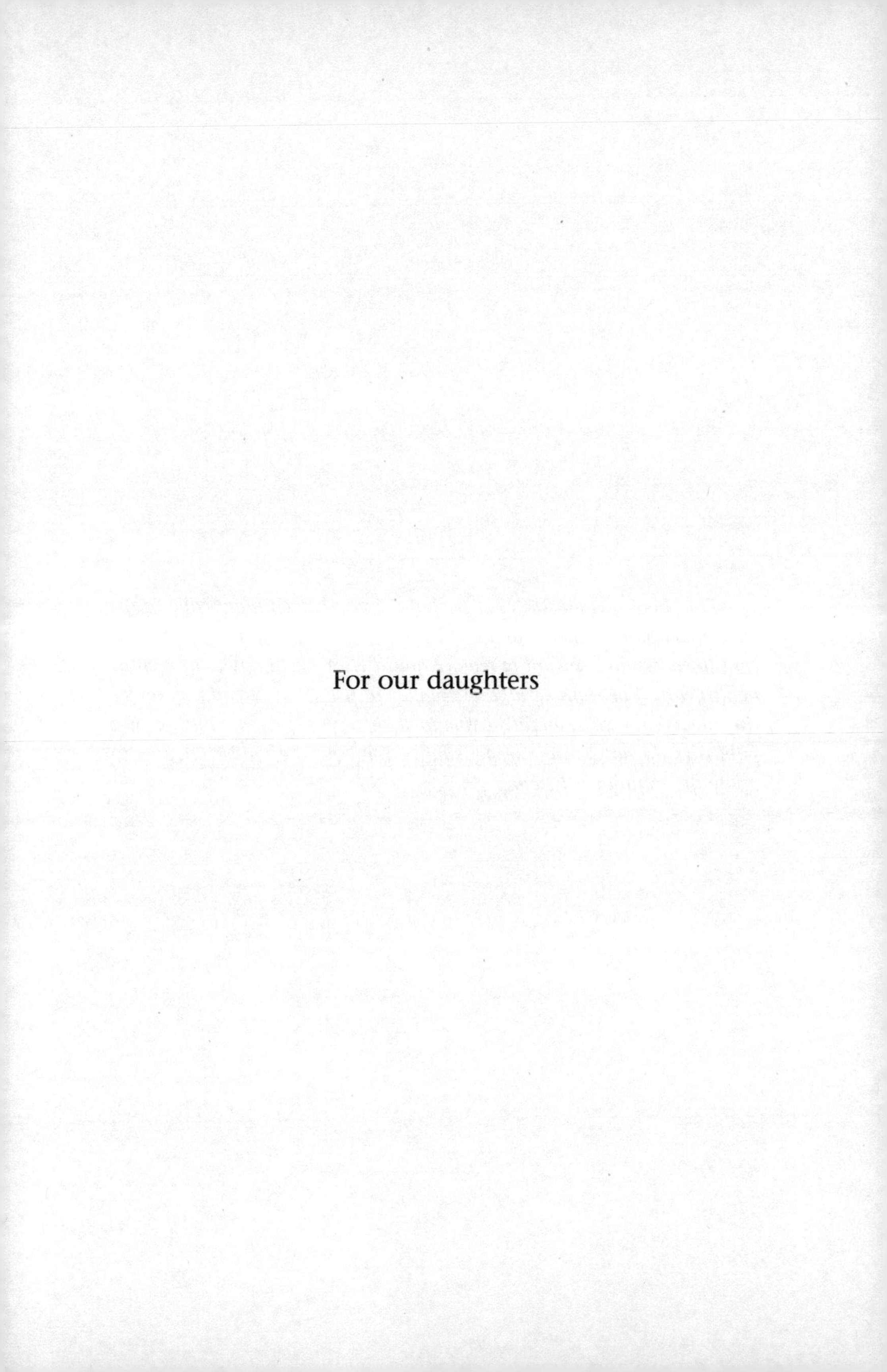
For our daughters

This book demonstrates a personal growth technique called tapping. It is not a substitute for psychiatric care or psychotherapy. Nothing contained herein is meant to replace qualified medical advice or mental health care. The authors urge the reader to use these techniques under the supervision of a qualified therapist or physician. The author and publisher do not assume responsibility for how the reader chooses to apply the techniques herein.

CONTENTS

FOREWORD

An almost-lived life is the greatest of tragedies. We've all known people who have fabulous potential, yet never turn it into reality.

I've talked to many people as they were near the ends of their lives. One, my former neighbor Janice, was in her late eighties. She lived with her husband, Bill, who was just hitting ninety and in declining health. Conversations with Janice were peppered with her regrets over missed opportunities, carelessly discarded chances to live life fully, visions of what might have been, and the bitter realization that she and Bill would never be able to make up for lost time.

You don't want to end up like Janice and Bill. Seize every opportunity to release your blocks and claim your potential. Tomorrow will not be a better day to start growing. Fulfillment is not going to be easier down the road. There's never going to be a better time than now to reach for transformation. The day we start taking action is the day we start maximizing our potential.

Margaret and David's book is a marvelous guide to finding and releasing the blocks to that potential. Margaret, as one of today's leading coaches, and David, as a deeply discerning psychologist, provide insights, tools, and a systematic approach to clearing your blocks and realizing your full potential.

Margaret has found that her coaching clients have in common a lack of self-belief, even though many are high achievers. They use a microscope to enlarge their flaws, while shrinking their strengths and gifts. In *Unblocked,* she and David provide a step-by-step map to seeing yourself clearly and releasing the arguments—often buried deep in the subconscious—that stifle your potential.

The central transformational practice used in the book is Emotional Freedom Techniques or EFT, which is often called "tapping" because it uses fingertip tapping on acupuncture points to balance the body's energy system. It also includes elements of two well-researched psychological methods, cognitive therapy and exposure therapy. Over 100 clinical trials demonstrating EFT's efficacy for everything from pain to depression to fibromyalgia can be found at Research.EFTuniverse.com. EFT is particularly effective in treating conditions arising from traumatic memories, such as PTSD.

In one EFT workshop, I tapped with "Colonel Chuck," a veteran who had served as a marine pilot during the Vietnam war. Chuck's worst memory was of his first solo flight off the deck of an aircraft carrier. Just as his Super Sabre jet became airborne, the control tower operator yelled, "Engine fire! Get out!" Chuck was just high enough above the waves to eject safely. But this and other combat traumas led him to develop PTSD. On a scale of 0 to 10, Chuck's emotion around the event was a 10—and that was more than forty years after the accident.

Chuck and I tapped on the operator's words, on the flames he saw when he looked behind him, and other aspects of the event. Chuck's numbers began to drop. Eventually, he was at a 0. He took a very deep breath and said, "I'm grateful I survived." In psychology that's called a "cognitive shift," because it indicates a major change in mental perspective. Chuck went from trembling with fear as he told the story to gratitude for having survived the threat.

A meta-analysis of six studies of EFT for PTSD found it had astoundingly large treatment effects. On the most common scale used to measure the effect of a psychological treatment, 2 indicates a measurable effect. Five represents a moderate effect, while a score of 8 means that the treatment produces large effects. The analysts found that the effect size for EFT was 29. That's completely off the charts. And it didn't take long to treat those PTSD patients effectively: between 4 and 10 treatment sessions. That's how quickly and effectively tapping can turn the fears that block our potential into the strengths that propel us forward.

With focus, effort, and practice, we can change dysfunctional thoughts and behaviors that lie at the level of conscious awareness. If you're habitually late, you can train yourself to be on time. If you have a habit of throwing your dirty socks on the sofa, the objections of your partner might lead you to discipline yourself to toss them in the laundry instead. But that's the level of personal change that most of us can accomplish without outside help.

Subconscious patterns are a much greater challenge. We can't access them directly. We often need outside help—whether this book, an online course, or a practitioner—to even identify them. Unless we get that help, these patterns can block us from fulfilling our dreams our whole life long, and we wind up like Janice and Bill.

Margaret describes the pain she feels as she witnesses people repeating such patterns of suffering year after year. David reminds us that our bodies remember early childhood insults that our minds do not. These subconscious somatic instructions can keep us rooted in maladaptive behaviors at odds with our conscious goals. We can't do things that are clearly good for us, and we can't understand why.

That's because the source of these impulses is deep below the surface. *Unblocked* helps bring them to consciousness, where we can recognize and work on them. Unless we do so, they may surface involuntarily—as compulsions, addictions, chronic self-sabotage, or uncomfortable emotions. Margaret and David remind us that while these patterns may show up in our marriages, workplaces, and social interactions, they are rooted in early childhood.

Surprisingly, many of them were adaptive when we were little. Dissociation, for instance, can serve as an essential coping mechanism for a child. Trapped in a dysfunctional family, dissociation allows a child to "forget" bad events. This allows her to continue to function in a situation from which there is no escape.

Though behaviors like dissociation are adaptive at the time, they have an expiration date. When we're still using dissociation as adults, that date is long past. We've failed to claim our present-day power. The essential work of adulthood is healing our childhood wounds so that we can reclaim the full range of our potential.

Margaret shows how tapping gives us a safe way to approach the traumatic events of our past as empowered adults.

Healing the chakra system through EFT helps energy move through our bodies in a healthy rather than distorted way. We might feel uncomfortable energy surges when this first happens, but Margaret reassures us that these internal upheavals are simply the result of energy that's been locked in our bodies since childhood moving freely at last.

Margaret and David emphasize the importance of starting at the root chakra, which has to do with safety and security. They note that many self-help addicts start at the top chakras, those in the head. They seek to change their mind-set, use positive affirmations, or pursue spiritual enlightenment.

Margaret and David help us realize that unless our foundation is solid, it will continue to undermine these lofty aspirations. That's why they start by addressing the survival fears and self-doubt that lurk in the lower energy centers.

Case histories drawn from Margaret's extensive work with a wide variety of clients vividly illustrate the obstacles and potentials of this approach. One example is a professional woman climbing the corporate ladder but racked with internal self-doubt. Margaret traced the adult symptoms to childhood experiences of being unsupported.

In other case histories, people feel they have to earn their right to feel safe, every day, by vigilantly following the rules of being perfect or successful. Old childhood scripts can also show up as overwork, poor boundaries, low self-esteem, poor body image, perfectionism, procrastination, being an unfulfilled super-achiever, and other maladies.

Unblocked contains a whole series of practical "Healing Experiences." These chapters will have you tapping, as well as uncovering all the possible psychological and childhood obstacles that hold you back. They combine Margaret's chakra framework with David's psychoanalytic approach in a complementary synthesis. Both are entry points into the hidden world that lies below the conscious mind.

The weekly homework gives structure to your transformational journey. Vivid visualizations provide the words to reshape your experience, layer after layer. You'll journal, listen intently to your body, feel your emotions, install new habits, tap away stress, and unfold a new vision of yourself at your own perfect pace.

Powerful and detailed tapping scripts approach healing from many angles. The Healing Experiences also contain links to additional video content to support and accelerate your progress from healing to empowerment.

Unblocked is a unique combination of Eastern energy work and the insights of Western psychology. Clear and compelling, this book's systematic approach will help you find the obstacles that have been holding you back, and clear them. As your wise and compassionate guides, Margaret and David will take you on a transformational journey to your full potential. The adventure beckons!

— Dawson Church, award winning author of *Bliss Brain: The Neuroscience of Remodeling Your Brain for Resilience, Creativity, and Joy*

INTRODUCTION

THE FUN-HOUSE MIRROR

Imagine a friend comes to stay at your house for the first time. All is going well until you show her where the bathroom is, and she freaks out. "Is this a joke? What the hell kind of mirror is this?"

You quickly check your reflection and see exactly what you always see every day. "It looks completely fine to me," you say, bewildered. "Same as always!"

But your friend is unconvinced. She rifles through her bag, pulls out her hand mirror, and holds it up to your face. What you see in her mirror takes your breath away. You see a face you barely recognize. A face with beautiful, smart, kind eyes; lovely skin; and a beaming smile full of life.

What is this magic? you wonder. *Surely it's a trick.* But it is no trick. It is just the first time you are seeing *you*, beholding yourself as you truly are. And you are incredibly, almost unimaginably, beautiful.

Your surge of joy at seeing this truth suddenly mixes with shock as you look back at your lifelong mirror. Another truth emerges—the truth about your old mirror. You see it now for the damaged, fun-house mirror it has always been. With newly awakened eyes, you clearly see the distortions that make some of your features appear grossly huge and others weirdly tiny. You can't help but notice the huge black flecks hiding entire sections of your face.

Comparing your reflection in the two mirrors is overwhelming. Tears flow as you take stock of the lifetime of pain this mirror has needlessly caused you, from the shame of believing you are somehow flawed to all the ways those beliefs have stopped you from living fearlessly with full-on joy and passion.

"All this time I thought I was ugly, not good enough, broken," you whisper. "But it was never true. I have always been beautiful—inside and out."

A WORLD FULL OF NEEDLESS PAIN

One of the most difficult experiences for me (Margaret) is to see people walking around with so much needless pain on every level: emotionally, mentally, physically, and spiritually. Even those who, from the outside looking in, have successful lives struggle with emotional pain, whether in the form of self-doubt and anxiety or powerlessness and regret. Many people play it small, feel invisible, isolate, or are afraid to show up in life for fear of making a mistake or not being "good enough." Others take big steps toward their goals and dreams only to sabotage their efforts when on the cusp of success. A common theme for many people is working tremendously hard to prove they are worthy of taking up space on this planet. Yet somehow, despite all they accomplish, they never feel good enough on the inside.

Even as a child, I wanted to "fix" my classmates as we all began to struggle with insecurities, which usually revolved around feeling ugly or embarrassed about hair, clothes, and acne. Much like in the fun-house mirror story, it was as if they were seeing an exaggerated version of their imperfections and none of their beauty.

But no matter how hard I tried to convince my friends of what I could see—that they were beautiful, smart, funny, amazing, and had nothing to worry about—I couldn't change what they saw. I tried passion. I tried logic. I tried humor. And I tried tears. Their inner beliefs always won, and over the years, I watched how those insecurities showed up in their body language, confidence, choices, and actions. By high school I had decided that you can't change people on the inside, so I followed the family footsteps and became an engineer.

For 18 years I worked as a chemical engineer at several Fortune 500 companies. I was promoted many times because I seemed to have a gift for mentoring and managing people, and I brought home a nice paycheck. From the outside looking in, I was secure and successful. But I never really felt passionate about my career or the work itself.

With the birth of my daughter at age 30, I moved into less stressful roles, taking technical sales positions that paid well and let me work from a home office. Cushy, yes, but I was bored, uninspired, and mailing it in. *Aren't I meant to do something more?* I would ask myself often. *Something bigger?*

Then one day I saw the great author and speaker Wayne Dyer on TV talking about the power of intention. Suddenly everything changed. He seemed to be speaking directly to me. "Yes, Margaret, you are meant to do something more—find it!"

After arguing with Wayne in my head for a week, I took the leap and set off to completely change my career path. I found myself leaning back into my childhood calling to help others change and heal. I got certified in hypnotherapy and Emotional Freedom Technique (EFT), a clinically proven energy-psychology intervention also known as tapping. I was convinced that if I could just help people clear out their erroneous thinking—the distortions in their mirror—they would see what I could see: their beauty, gifts, and worthiness.

NAVIGATING MY NEW PATH

In my early 40s, I started seeing clients, and I was eager to help them with my new techniques. Most of my first clients were curious about tapping for specific issues. They wanted help eliminating fears over public speaking, alleviating physical issues that started as emotional issues, and reducing food cravings so they could lose weight. But as I started to market myself more and more to entrepreneurs and career-driven people, the work got more complex.

On the surface they wanted help reaching their goals, and I promised to help them clear away whatever was holding them back. Their complaints were common enough. Most came under the heading of anxiety over doing something, such as dreading a confrontation with their boss or subordinates, panic over giving a self-promoting presentation, or apprehension about a court case or negotiation. Or they felt stuck in a dead-end job or at a level of earning potential. Many clients suffered from procrastination and had trouble taking important steps toward their goals and dreams, which often meant they were self-limiting their success and income.

All of these people came to work with me because they recognized that they were the source of their problems, usually saying some version of "It's me! I sabotage myself." The more clients I worked with, the more I saw that underneath all the anxiety, procrastination, and "stuckness" were bigger issues. When it came down to it, we always got to a familiar and similar place: Secretly, they questioned whether they were good enough to take their next steps. These folks lacked the courage and confidence that come with believing in yourself.

Tapping positively and immediately impacted stress and anxiety levels. For some clients it was like an instant miracle. But for those who felt the most stuck, the standard use of tapping wasn't getting to the heart of their issues. There was a deeper side to their self-doubt that seemed truer and more certain to them than the gifts, talents, and potential that I could clearly see. Here I was again, standing in front of a mirror with incredibly smart, talented, and big-hearted people who saw clear evidence of their flaws and only glimmers of their light. No wonder they were procrastinating!

The truth is I was keenly aware of struggling with the exact same doubts as I tried to grow my coaching business, so I knew what they were going through. This was a crossroads for me. I realized that escaping this stuckness was bigger than what any technique could offer and that helping people move past this was exactly what I had always felt called to do. I became determined to find a way to create a major shift in how my clients felt about and believed in themselves. I wanted them (as well as myself) to have the confidence, passion, and courage to take action. I had to figure this out!

I put on my engineer thinking cap and doubled down on my working theory: every outer problem, struggle, or complaint has an inner root cause. I had great tools, but I needed to shape what I was doing into a system of getting consistent and more far-reaching results. I focused all my studies and client work on figuring out *how* I could get people to change. I became obsessed with the *how*.

Stacks of books on the subject focused on using willpower or affirmations or on the "mental gymnastics" of trying not to think negative thoughts. They all boiled down to the one message I was trying to get to the bottom of: "You have to stop doubting yourself! Believe in yourself!" But their *hows* seemed to scratch the surface of change. I needed something that went much deeper.

It wasn't until I started learning about the chakra system (the body's seven energy centers) that I felt the start of something big. As far as I was concerned, I had suddenly found a treasure map to healing.

FROM *HOW* TO *WHERE*

Through studying the chakras and using what I learned experimentally in client sessions, I gathered that the roots of self-doubt were in secret, guarded, long-forgotten places. These were places that clients either could not show me or were consciously or unconsciously leading me away from with lots of distracting details. But in understanding the chakras, I now had a map guiding me to *where* I had to go to get to the root of an issue.

All along I had been asking the wrong question. Instead of asking *how* to help people shift, I needed to focus on the *where*. *Where* do I need to go to solve these inner problems? *Where* are they rooted? By changing the question, I began to crack the code to getting bigger changes and bigger results.

I learned where to dig deep to get to the inner root causes of self-doubt and fear that lie beneath procrastination, perfectionism, and self-sabotage. I crafted methods to safely and compassionately take clients to these places where we could introduce tapping to heal in unexpected ways. I watched as, step by step, healing those places in my clients was like removing blocks to their natural self-belief and self-love and allowing confidence, joy, and passion to rise through their system.

After these sessions clients were happier, bolder, more enthusiastic, and in action. They felt empowered!

A remarkable number of client e-mails, phone calls, and sessions started with the giddy words, "Margaret, you are never going to believe what I did. . . ." These words were usually followed by tales of moments when they surprised themselves (and often those around them) by doing something big with a new level of ease and enthusiasm. Those clients honored me with their trust by allowing me to lead them to their innermost spaces of pain and fear. They challenged me to better navigate where to go to get meaningful change.

Like any good engineer, I then put my methods and discoveries into a systematic, step-by-step approach that anyone can learn and get seemingly impossible results from even when using it on their own. And all it takes is two fingertips, a commitment to go through the program, and a desire to feel more empowered than ever.

All this talk about tapping and chakras might be sounding a bit too woo-woo for some of you. If you're feeling skeptical, stick with me anyway, because you don't need to buy into this for it to work. You only need to try it and feel what happens.

WHAT EXACTLY ARE THE CHAKRAS?

The energetic system of the chakras stems from ancient Hindu yogic tradition. Centuries ago yogis compartmentalized the body's functioning into seven major energy centers that are known today in the West as the Root, Sacral, Solar Plexus, Heart, Throat, Third Eye, and Crown Chakras.

Responsible for the quality of our physical bodies, feelings and emotions, agency, ability to love, creativity, spirituality, and mind, the chakras sum up the human experience. They are pure energy assets designed to bring us vibrancy, joy, confidence, passion, worthiness, and empowerment.

A Rainbow of Energy

Each chakra is responsible for powering a different level of human existence and is associated with a color of the rainbow.

1. The Root Chakra is red and represents safety and security.
2. The Sacral Chakra is orange and represents creativity.
3. The Solar Plexus Chakra is yellow and represents self-esteem and willpower.
4. The Heart Chakra is green and represents wisdom, love, and compassion.
5. The Throat Chakra is blue and represents communication.
6. The Third Eye Chakra is indigo and represents intuition and imagination.
7. The Crown Chakra is violet and represents higher consciousness.

In *Anatomy of the Spirit*, author Caroline Myss writes about the seven chakras as stages of personal and spiritual power. At each chakra level, we gain more energy—more power—and become conscious about how to use it.

Each chakra carries a unique gift of energy—a unique level of consciousness that develops at specific ages. The Root Chakra, for instance, begins to form as soon as we are born. It's designed to help us feel solid and grounded in the physical world. By the time we reach adolescence, we're opening up to our imagination and self-reflection at the sixth chakra, or the Third Eye Chakra. In adulthood we're finally able to open our Crown Chakra of enlightenment and see possibilities for ourselves far beyond our family paradigm.

How we experience life during these developmental periods when our chakras are unfolding will either nurture our chakras' natural rising energy that is so core to being an empowered, happy adult—or block it.

In the foreword to *Anatomy of the Spirit,* author C. Norman Shealy, M.D., Ph.D., calls the chakras regulators of life-energy flow: "The major biological batteries of your emotional biography." If even one chakra is blocked, some of our power is blocked, and life will feel less joyful. We will feel as if we have been denied certain natural, inalienable birthrights. Fulfilling our purpose becomes a struggle.

In this context I see chakras as a brilliant map of the whole of human consciousness.

BLOCKED CHAKRAS

As energy rises from chakra to chakra, it influences the other chakras. The strength of the fourth chakra (the Heart Chakra) is dependent upon the strength of the first, second, and third chakras. Enlightenment (the seventh chakra) requires the energy of all the lower six chakras. Although they are interconnected and interdependent, each chakra has a unique mission to fulfill, and it all starts at the foundation, or the Root Chakra.

In a perfect world, the chakras develop fully and freely, their energy allowed to course throughout the body uninterrupted. In an imperfect world that at times teaches us we're unworthy, unimportant, powerless, or unlovable, those wounds and beliefs act to block and misdirect chakra energy and therefore our personal power. If we truly believe, for instance, that we are undeserving of earning more money, we hold back on the rising energy that would compel us to confidently ask for a raise. We work hard and wonder why we can't seem to get ahead, much less make ends meet. This type of struggle is a symptom of a blocked chakra.

Technically, the chakras are always opening and closing depending on what's happening in any given moment and what kind of energy we allow to flow through that space. So a blocked chakra doesn't necessarily mean a closed chakra. When imagining a blocked chakra, think in terms of how big the channel of energy is. Some of us have a sliver of energy running up through the chakras. What we're going for is more volume—the stuff of fire-hose energy.

The cost of blocked chakra energy is enormous. Blocked chakras can limit us to a life of pain, disappointment, unfulfilled dreams, depression, anxiety, addiction, disease, and other woes. Some of my clients avoided relationships for many years because they didn't trust themselves to set boundaries. Others were stuck in jobs they felt no passion for because they followed what was expected of them instead of listening to their inner voice. Still others left a job or relationship only to feel lost and unsure of who they were or what they really wanted.

Free-flowing chakras empower us. Chakras blocked by fear, guilt, shame, and a host of other barriers, render us powerless. The bulk of this pain resides in the lower chakras.

THE MESSY LOWER CHAKRAS

The chakras are divided into upper and lower halves, with the Heart Chakra—the seat of wisdom—in the middle. The upper chakras (Crown, Third Eye, and Throat) are our sources of creativity, inspiration, and enlightenment. Because they are spiritual in nature, they have always been somewhat glorified in the pursuit of higher consciousness. The lower chakras (Solar Plexus, Sacral, and Root) are the bases of our power and responsible for how safe we feel to express our authentic selves in this world. They offer what I call empowerment energy.

Empowerment energy is the surge that lifts us into acting on inspired thoughts and following through. It's full of courage, deservedness, worthiness, and certainty, and we know it when we feel it. It is internal and a birthright. Using it feels good and right and meant to be because when we exercise empowerment energy, we do it the spirit of everyone's highest good. Empowerment energy is capable of effecting momentous change. It's hard, even painful, not to act on this energy. Denying it leads to suffering.

Empowerment energy is different than power, which is usually an energy we use over others—such as a parent's power over their young children or a boss's power over an employee. This kind of power comes from position and so depends on external circumstances. The "good" parent or boss uses their power wisely, but many people abuse this type of power. It's impossible to abuse empowerment energy, which comes not from ego or position but from our very core.

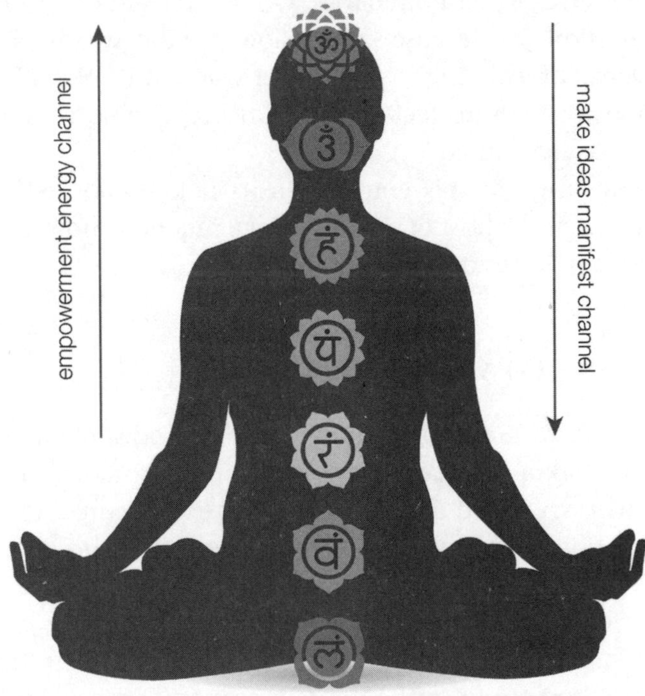

Figure 1

Empowerment energy (see figure 1) starts at the Root Chakra and flows upward. Manifestation (having an idea and turning it into a reality) starts at the Crown and works its way down. Struggling to manifest our dreams is a sign that lower chakra energy is blocked, because most of the practical work involved in making dreams come true happens in the lower chakras. For example, we may have a great idea to open a bakery but never come up with the down payment necessary to buy or rent the building. Releasing blocked empowerment energy is our focus in this book.

The lower chakras are messier than the upper chakras. They harbor the roots of complicated emotions of such as fear, guilt, and shame. They involve long-forgotten memories and distant events that shaped us as children. When they are blocked, it means we are filled with fear, pain, trauma, and all the things we don't like about ourselves. This blockage is compounded in the powerful Heart Chakra. When we lean into these four chakras, each lights the way to secret, guarded, forgotten spaces that hold the roots to our biggest struggles. These are sacred spaces *where* the real healing takes place, and where big transformation happens. And it's where we're going to spend most of our time.

HEALING THE CHAKRAS

You might be well versed in chakraspeak. If you're not, no worries. You don't technically need to know much about them to heal them. It's kind of like recovering from a cold. You don't have to understand how the body suddenly turns on its healing mechanism. You just need to know you've got a virus and then understand how to take care of the symptoms: drink plenty of clear fluids, get plenty of rest, and maybe take some extra vitamin C, and before you know it you feel better.

Likewise, with the chakras, you just need to know that something is off and then take care of the symptoms, which often include behaviors such as procrastination and self-sabotage, by following the process in this book. I will guide you through the lower chakras as you tap while reading a script, visualize, cry or yawn a bit every now and then (that's how you know you're unblocking energy), tap some more, and you will feel better and then stronger and more empowered than ever.

Still, it's good to have some understanding of the powers that lie within each of your chakras. Plenty of books on the market describe the intricacies of the chakras in detail. (One of my favorites is *Eastern Body, Western Mind* by Anodea Judith.) In *Unblocked* I give you enough information to get to know your chakras as I have interpreted them through my many years of working with clients. Throughout most of this book, however, you'll be focused on a process of healing them—on opening up the natural flow of energy that's been blocked over the years.

THE OTHER SIDE OF THE TRACKS: DAVID'S STORY

Like Margaret, from an early age I also wanted to help people. By the time I was 17, I was a certified emergency medical technician and the youngest member of my local first aid squad. "Beyond my years" at that still-tender age, I was skilled at intervening at the scene of motor vehicle accidents, providing life support to people in cardiac arrest, and attending to physical injuries from the minor to the severe. But what made the most profound impression on me were the things I saw that I could do nothing about: the victims of the car accident who died before I got there; the terrified and grief-stricken faces of parents, partners, and children who watched helplessly as I carried their loved ones out on a stretcher; or that teenager (around my age) with whom I sat quietly in the back of the ambulance on the way to the hospital following his overdose.

What took hold of me then were two of the most basic existential questions: *Why did these things happen? How do you live in a world where such horrible things happen?* It turned out that this was not a passing phase of teenage angst but a defining moment—a turning-inward that took root in me and has since guided my journey into the present day. This exposure to external, bodily trauma forced my attention toward the inner world; to what traumatic experiences of various shapes and sizes do to our insides; and to how our outer experiences shape and sometimes shatter our sense of self, others, and the world. At the time I was not sure why, but I needed to make sense of that for myself and others.

So I set upon a course to study the invisible wounds for which there weren't words—the hidden fractures and heartbreaks that lived silently in the shadows. I could sense these wounds in the people around me and was dimly aware of them in myself, but they called to me as a mysterious presence that I felt close to and needed to understand.

My doctoral training in clinical psychology was all about this, as was my formal training in psychoanalysis that followed. I studied when, where, and how the mind and heart bend and break. And I examined closely those forces that shape us into who we are, along with the many forms of psychotherapy that attempt to heal internal wounds, promote growth, and free us up to live a fuller life.

By the time I met my wife and co-author, it had been 20 years since I sat with my first patient, a survivor of trauma whose parting gift of a framed photograph of a street in Rome remains perched on my office desk as I write these words. When I met Margaret, I was well established in private practice and held teaching roles in academic institutions and leadership positions in clinical settings. I had trained at one of Harvard's prestigious teaching hospitals and had been supervised by some of the best and brightest minds on the planet. And with all of that under my belt, I had come to the same humble conclusion that the psychiatrist Harry Stack Sullivan sounded out decades earlier: "We are all much more simply human than otherwise."

The human predicament is something we all share, and the workings of the mind warrant humble reverence from whatever angle we approach them. In other words I didn't have all the answers, and the established traditions in which I was schooled didn't have a monopoly on anything. Anchored and disciplined in them as I was, I knew intuitively that other models of the human experience and treatment modalities also had much to offer. But when Margaret and I met, she knew only that I was a clinical psychologist and psychoanalyst—and she was scared.

Though Margaret couldn't help but speak passionately about her work and her involvement with tapping, chakras, and energy psychology, she also braced herself. As I listened quietly, she anticipated judgment and dismissal by this academically trained Ph.D., only to find that I embraced it all. She was surprised to learn that I was no stranger to alternative healing modalities and had done some of my own healing work in the human-energy field with a student of Barbara Brennan (author of *Hands of Light*). Professionally, my clinical work with trauma of various kinds had also required me to reach beyond traditional psychotherapy so I could better accompany my patients through their healing process. So by the time Margaret and I met, I had already experimented with and critically examined many alternative healing modalities—some of which I rejected completely on scientific grounds (for lacking conceptual coherence and empirical validity), whereas others I remained quite open to because of their demonstrated efficacy.

Margaret's systematic approach to integrating the chakra system (a grounding and guiding conceptual framework) with tapping (a clinically proven technique) and guided exposure through visualization (another clinically proven technique) felt like a breath of fresh air for this practicing therapist. For me, Margaret's creative and integrative blend of several elements fills a gap in traditional forms of psychotherapy and gets at some of the places where we are blocked internally that we might otherwise have no other way of accessing.

Fast-forwarding several years, here we are, and my contribution as co-author and commentator of this book represents another embrace of Margaret and her work. My commentaries in the chapters ahead will provide support to Margaret's ideas and guided tapping processes by drawing upon scientific disciplines whose accumulated wisdom and empirically validated research have anchored me during the past 20 years of my clinical practice.

Margaret's approach may engage the inner skeptic in some readers. I have much respect and appreciation for this part of any of us. Who we are and where we come from are matters too important to get wrong, and speculation about them runs counter to our project of establishing a more empowered foundation on which to stand within ourselves. So, from my inner skeptic to yours, I hope that the robust research findings in the fields of childhood development, attachment, and treatment outcome research help to establish trust that Margaret's approach stands on solid ground.

Finally, my commentaries are intended to speak to readers like me who are also practicing psychotherapists or mental health counselors. My words are intended to serve as a bridge between frames of reference familiar to a psychotherapist and Margaret's work. I continue to discover and marvel at the many points of contact between these two cultures of healing, and I hope that some of the ideas I put forth are useful to you as you transition into and traverse between Margaret's model and those more familiar to you.

MARGARET'S ADVICE FOR HOW TO USE THIS PROGRAM

Unblocked is divided into four parts, each with four chapters. Each part focuses on one of the four lower chakras—the empowerment energy chakras. The first chapter in each part is the setup chapter. It introduces the basics of a chakra—what it's responsible for, how it gets blocked, how much this blockage has cost us, and what you can look forward to when its energy is flowing once again.

Each of the remaining three chapters in each part are devoted to a Healing Experience. This is where you get your hands dirty and even start rolling in the mud, so to speak.

My co-author, David Raniere, Ph.D., is my husband. He's also a brilliant psychologist and psychoanalyst who has been trained to use tapping in his clinical practice. He has been a sounding board, guiding presence, and major influence in my work. At the end of each setup chapter, he explains why and how the Healing

Experiences work, validating not only the tapping process but also the importance of chakra work.

In the Healing Experience chapters, you'll always start with a visualization that takes you to the *where*—the specific places and times in your life that you need to visit to make real and lasting change. I sometimes ask you to "feel into" the experience. This is simply my way of asking you to be fully present for at least a few seconds. Each visualization is followed with a tapping script that guides you through voicing, releasing, and calming intense emotions and even old, unquestioned beliefs while you tap on acupressure points (see figure 2). The intention is to open, engage, and release unconscious thoughts and beliefs that are holding you down.

Each Healing Experience chapter ends with a Next Steps section. These include exercises to free up even more energy as well as suggestions for how to practice your new skills. They will help you to keep tapping and chakra work in the forefront of your daily existence.

TIMELINE: HOW LONG DOES IT TAKE?

How quickly you get through the book is up to you—sort of. Some of you might find it tempting to dash through all the Healing Experiences in the interest of, well, healing quickly. But I recommend going at a pace that *feels* right to you.

I offer some guidance about when you might want to keep going through a script before moving on, but you will want to listen to your inner guidance as well. It's not uncommon to spend days or weeks tapping on one script—or returning to it multiple times—while breezing through other scripts.

Likewise, the Next Steps sections can be done at your own pace. I suggest doing each Next Step for a week, but that's just a guideline. For some people a week is enough time to dig deep and realize how many opportunities there are to tap and unblock empowerment energy.

Although you get to decide how much time to spend on a Next Step, script, or chakra, be aware that procrastination and self-sabotage (two common signs of blocked empowerment energy) may be at play. If you find yourself making excuses for why you can't get to the work or putting it off for weeks or months, you might want to map out a schedule for yourself or tell yourself you will just do one script today. Be kind to yourself and plow through it if you must. I promise you will not regret it.

VISUALIZATION: A DOOR TO THE UNCONSCIOUS

Throughout the Healing Experiences, I will ask you to close your eyes and picture different times in your life—some from the past and some in the future. You will use your imagination to visit that time by simply allowing an image to form in your mind. Guided visualization is not meant to calm but instead to uncover and activate chakra-specific blocks. We are looking to intentionally trigger strong emotions and the negative beliefs that accompany them.

Visualization allows us to get impressions from our unconscious instead of from what we consciously think or remember. We will do this before, during, and after tapping, as if peeling an onion layer by layer. The visualizations I guide you through are important because they are an effective means of hearing from the emotional, illogical, and primitive unconscious mind—a storehouse of first (and second) chakra information that is beyond our conscious awareness and even memory. We may not be cognizant of what's in the storehouse, but it holds the invisible roots to what we need to heal.

Sigmund Freud, the founder of psychoanalysis, viewed the unconscious as a part of the mind that holds impulses, wishes, desires (including those that are learned to be socially unacceptable), traumatic memories, and emotions we actively try not to feel. Sometimes, unbeknownst to us, a battle erupts between a conscious desire or goal and our unconscious that registers the goal as threatening, dangerous, or something that, if achieved, will be somehow painful. We struggle to act or follow through with a plan, but we don't know why. We are unaware of the pain, trauma, or danger that our unconscious associates with our exciting new plans. We're acting based on a hidden agenda of which we are unaware.

Whether good, bad, right, wrong, true, or false, this lifetime of data remains in our unconscious mind to this day but is difficult to access directly. We might get a glimpse of them in dreams or unexpectedly voice one in a "Freudian slip." (But we can—and will—use tapping to get to them.) It's as if we collected this data, put it in our storage box, and threw away the key.

Closing the eyes and visiting these important places by allowing the mind to imagine a picture full of details, feelings, and impressions can result in stunning amounts of information that illuminate the healing we need to do. This is true even for those who feel initially skeptical about what their imagination is conjuring up. So as you follow the instructions to visualize a person or event taking shape, resist the temptation to overthink it. Because the unconscious is not ruled by logic or the linear progression of time—but instead seems to operate in strong emotions, metaphors, and pictures—we must trust that what appears in our mind's eye means something important to us.

The historical accuracy of what we may picture is of little importance. We're going for the powerful emotions and meanings that reveal how the past has created the present.

Visualization also allows us to do something I find incredibly powerful as a practitioner and results-oriented person: After going through a round of tapping, we can check in and get an instant measure on the impact and progress of the healing work by comparing our pre- and post-tapping visualizations. Each time the picture in our mind's eye will have shifted. This new picture with new information shows us where we are in the process and the next important set of emotions and meanings to work on.

For example, if the imagined picture has become more intense emotionally, that tells us we have hit on something that needs more attention. Has the emotion shifted from intense fear to sadness or anger? That tells us which emotion to shift to voicing and honoring with the next tapping round. Does the child we are imagining now seem happy and content and to know we are there instead of terrified and alone? That's a sign of healing.

Healing takes place when we are ready to move into being with the entirety of a given experience and hold a new space of compassion and understanding for ourselves. Believe me when I say that you will know it when you get there.

TAPPING: A CLINICALLY PROVEN MIND-BODY TECHNIQUE

Throughout the Healing Experiences, you'll be using Emotional Freedom Technique (EFT), commonly known as tapping. This evidence-based, clinically proven intervention effectively reduces anxiety and the stress response in a measurable physiological way even within minutes of use. Developed in the 1980s by clinical psychologist Roger Callahan, and popularized in the 1990s by his student Gary Craig, it is often used to treat post-traumatic stress disorder (PTSD) safely, and it's currently taking the world by storm.

The technique involves light tapping with the fingertips on certain acupuncture points (see figure 2) while recalling specific experiences that trigger fears, anxiety, or stress. The tapping acts like a physical switch, turning down the nervous system's fight-flight-freeze response within minutes of use. Because all intense, reactionary, and painful emotions have fear as a major element, tapping is a perfect mind-body tool to use with chakras, which are linked to the nervous system.

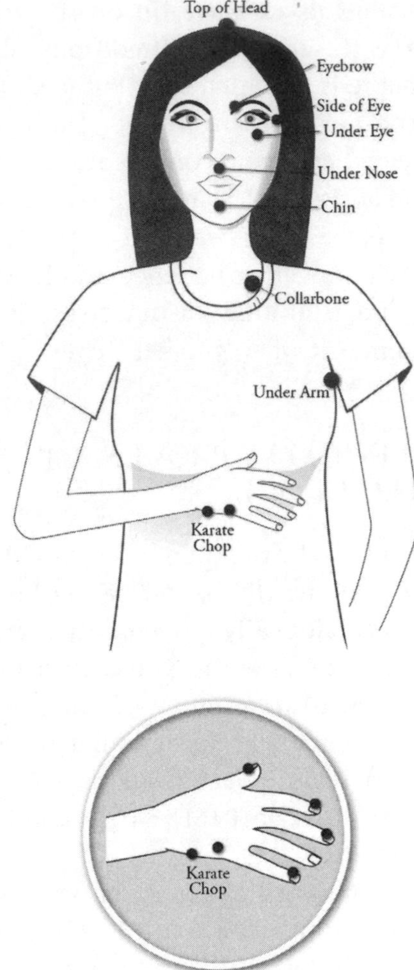

Figure 2

At the same time, tapping has been proven to stimulate, or switch on, the relaxation response, which is associated with many positive benefits from boosting the immune system to improving mental clarity and decision making. When used expertly EFT can produce *lasting* change, especially when paired with the tapping scripts provided in the Healing Experience chapters in this book.

I usually start tapping at the eyebrow points (see figure 2) and work my way down to the temples, below the eyes, below the nose, on the chin, on the collarbone, under the arms, on the hands, and then back up to the crown of the head. Tapping on any given point is optional. If you prefer not to tap under the arms or on the hands, for instance, so be it!

You can also begin and end your tapping on any point you want. Early practitioners of EFT followed a certain tapping order, but we've since learned that the order doesn't matter. It won't affect your outcome. Do whatever is most comfortable. You can use one hand and two fingers (index and middle) or two hands and four fingers so you are tapping on both sides of the body simultaneously. (You only need two fingers when tapping under the nose and on the chin—and one hand when tapping the opposite hand.)

Since the mid-1980s millions of people have used tapping safely at home by turning to videos, books, or experts featured on radio, television, or telesummits. One of the most popular online events, the Tapping World Summit, has been held annually since 2008 and attracts more than 2 million listeners.

Tapping has been proven overwhelmingly to be safe for self use by everyday people with everyday problems, even when experiencing strong emotions, because of the consistent calming effect it has on the nervous system. However, the *Unblocked* approach involves visualizations and tapping phrases that are meant to honestly voice strong emotions like fear, anger, and grief. There are times when intense emotions can come up quickly and/or unexpectedly as you tap through the process. If at any time, it begins to feel like too much or overwhelming during any of the visualizations or tapping contained in the Healing Experiences immediately pause and follow this protocol.

Protocol for Intense Emotional Reactions

Stop visualizing the scene that has triggered the intense emotions and stop using the words of the tapping script. Instead continue to tap silently as you breathe deeply and focus on your own breath as it flows in and out. For some people it's best to focus your attention on the sensation of your feet touching the floor and the chair supporting you as you breathe deeply. This will help you feel calm and grounded. For others it will feel better to physically get up and walk away from the process while you continue to tap silently and take full deep breaths. In that case, move your body, take a walk, shake it out, and swing your arms and intermittently stamp your feet to feel more grounded.

Next, listen to your body and reactions because they may be telling you this is too much to handle on your own and you don't need to do this alone or all at once. Reach out for support and discuss your reactions with a licensed mental health provider.

Contraindications for the Use of Tapping

There are emotional conditions and life circumstances for which tapping and/or tapping focused on activating strong emotions is either contraindicated or to be used only under the direct care of a mental health professional trained in this technique. A variety of psychological conditions involve significant difficulties regulating emotional states such that exposure to emotionally intense material can be overwhelming and have significantly adverse effects. In particular, individuals who suffer from dissociative disorders, impulse-control disorders, and panic disorder are advised to consult a mental health provider prior to utilizing this technique on their own. Tapping is also contraindicated for individuals suffering from borderline personality disorder, acute substance abuse, or for those who continue to be exposed to the traumatic experiences they wish to process, such that they are not in a sufficiently safe environment to process that trauma. Such conditions are best treated by licensed mental health providers. In addition, some psychological trauma can be too intense and emotionally painful to deal with on your own. If you have long-lasting or intense emotional or physical and/or sexual trauma it is essential that you consult your physician or a licensed mental health practitioner before using the Healing Experiences or tapping scripts in this book. Tapping is not a substitute for medical or mental health treatment.

TAPPING SCRIPTS: ENGAGING THE NERVOUS SYSTEM

Each Healing Experience chapter includes several tapping scripts designed to lead you to voice, hear, and honor all the pain, fear, and emotions triggered by each visualization. The words in these scripts invite you to dig deep, release the intensity of painful emotions, and charge up your empowerment energy.

The number of tapping scripts within each chapter varies, but you can repeat them as many times as you want if you feel you need more work. Text in the script is separated by dashes. This is your cue to move to the next tapping point (see figure 2). It's not essential that you move to the next point at that time. It's my way of ensuring you go through the tapping points at least once, and usually multiple times, during each script.

You'll want to read the scripts out loud as you tap. Sometimes I ask you to read them very loudly or even rant!

Every Healing Experience chapter includes a link to bonus content and discussion not contained in the book. Also, if you decide to purchase the audiobook, you'll have the added benefit of hearing me guide you through the tapping scripts and visualizations.

The content of the tapping scripts is based on years of working with clients. Many of the word choices are from the mouths of my clients and reflect common experiences. At times the words in the scripts might sound harsh and over-the-top and even feel wrong to say. Sometimes the only way to voice an injustice is to use the charged words of protest and outrage. So that's what we're going to do. (Whenever you read or listen to a script, make sure you tap at the same time. Reading these scripts without tapping might make you feel bad.) The idea is to voice, honor, and move stuck energy. I say that a lot in this book because it's a key process to unblocking chakra energy: voice, honor, and move.

Even though I sometimes ask you to say things to your parents, for instance, that you'd never dare utter, even in private, I promise you that no one gets hurt—not your loved ones, not your enemies, and certainly not you. You may go through some intense moments, but tapping ensures that you will always feel a sense of calm emotionally and physically. The longer you tap—even if you do so without saying a word—the greater the calm.

But getting calm is only part of the process. We will use tapping chakra by chakra to reclaim *you* and what you deserve to be, do, and have for your next chapter in life. I will guide you through the process, charging you up with the empowerment energy you need to create the life you want.

And please know that throughout the Healing Experiences, I'll be holding a space for you in my Heart Chakra—the chakra in which all healing takes place. Through my words and my belief in this process, I will, like a loving friend, hold your hand as you move forward into this uncharted, exciting, and *empowering* territory—and offer you a new mirror so you can behold your own incredible beauty and power.

This process of blending tapping with a systematic focus on the lower chakras to safely guide you to places you would never go on your own takes you directly to the hidden roots of your issues, expertly revealing blind spots, even to veteran tappers. The result is meaningful change that you can feel inside and see in your new words, actions, and enthusiasm. The promise is not just healing but *profound transformation in your personal power that changes the way you show up, speak, and act*!

Let's get started.

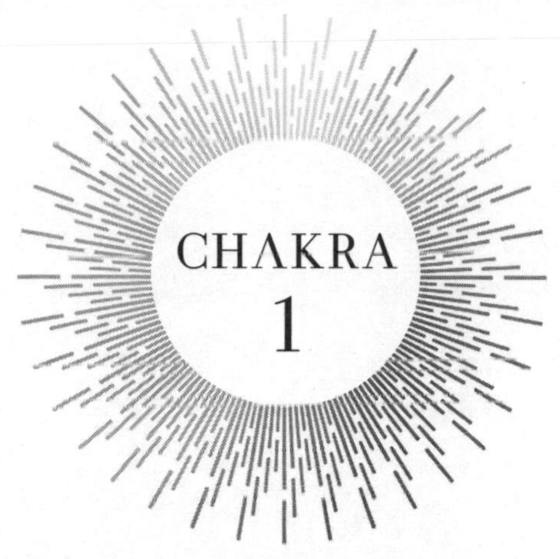

THE POWER OF PRESENCE—HEALING THE ROOT CHAKRA

Imagine . . . that your automatic,
unquestioned truth—
"*Of course I have the right*"—
calmed every whisper of self-doubt.

CHAPTER 1

RECLAIMING A GROUNDED, POWERFUL PRESENCE

In my many years of meeting with clients who want to make big changes in their lives but feel stuck, I've noticed a common denominator: Even without thinking about it in chakra terms, people tend to ignore the Root, or first, Chakra and go straight to the top—the upper chakras of mindset, positive affirmations, and enlightenment. If they are into personal growth, they meditate or practice yoga to clear the mind and become present and open. If they are more business focused, they set sizable goals, read mindset books, and try to think big and stay positive. But going to the top without doing the foundational work is like putting frosting on a moldy brownie—it looks good at first, but what's underneath eventually makes its way to the surface.

The gifts of the upper chakras are many, but they are very different from the lower-chakra empowerment energy gifts, which are required for real, underlying change. To own our power and rise to new challenges, we need to be present and grounded in a strong foundation of resiliency and self-belief. We need to address directly the not-so-positive sides of us instead of pretending they are not there. These tend to be the core, fear-based ways of operating that appear to work against us—the ones backed by thoughts such as *What if I am not good enough?*

These deep inner thoughts can fill us with anxiety and dread about doing the big things in life we dream about or even just taking the next step. We will experience scattered thinking, procrastination, and paralyzing perfectionism instead of the bold courage we need. Without a strong first chakra, our dreams and wishes can float untethered for years, as if in zero gravity, unable to gain traction. As one client said about the time she had lost: "And then a year became ten years, and I am running out of time."

Unblocking empowerment energy requires leaning into the difficult work of uncovering and transforming what stops us from boldly and confidently making our dreams happen. We need to find and clear the mold—the false beliefs and fears—that have been wired into our core since birth and are still running the show. We need to start at the bottom because the roots of our problems are in the Root Chakra.

Characteristics of the Root Chakra

Located at the bundle of nerves at the base of the spinal cord, the Root Chakra is where everything starts. The first chakra develops during infancy and childhood as part of the nervous system, which controls the physiological survival response known generally as *fight, flight, or freeze.* It also represents the body's first level of consciousness, which is a specialized awareness of ourselves as physical beings with safety and survival as the first order of importance. Because of the Root Chakra's connection to the physical, it is also known as the chakra of manifestation.

With a strong first chakra, we are standing on solid ground. Everything we do and everything we are feels supported. We have a powerful presence because we are comfortable in our skin. We generally feel safe, worthy, and self-empowered, knowing we can go for what we want with courage and resiliency. We are good at managing physical resources, opportunities, and wealth and rising up to meet challenges. People describe us as grounded and magnets for money, success, and luck.

The Root Chakra develops as we absorb and internalize our first tribe's (family's or caregiver's) beliefs and behaviors as our foundation of reality—the unquestioned "truths" about ourselves, our worthiness, the world, God, abundance, scarcity, and people. These early experiences form the foundation upon which the other six chakras (levels of consciousness) are built. The Root Chakra influences every other chakra and therefore everything we do.

FILLING THE FIRST CHAKRA CUP: SAFETY FIRST

Newborns may not look like they're thinking about life's big, heavy questions. But you might be surprised how much is going on in those cute little bodies. Already wired for safety and survival, an infant's nervous system has some pretty serious concerns, including: *Do I matter enough to be cared for and protected, to be loved? Am I important enough that my discomfort, pain, or hunger is noticed and attended to until it is soothed away?*

These are valid questions, given that infancy is a time when we are most vulnerable and completely dependent on our first tribe—our parents or other caregivers. It is as if our immature nervous system were asking the most basic of survival questions and our tribe were answering them.

Tribe

During infancy our tribe is our parents or other primary caregivers. Mom and Dad are God, responsible for ensuring we are nourished, kept warm and safe, and physically soothed when we feel anxious or agitated. Though eventually we will step into new tribes of people in schools, communities, and workplaces, we are born to trust and depend on our primary caregivers to teach us how to feel and act and what to expect from other people. They are either our safety net or the void inside where a securely felt safety net should be.

The infant nervous system constantly stands on alert for the answers to these survival questions. The consistent messages it receives are the raw biofeedback that influences the developing first chakra. Being lovingly held, soothed, and nourished in infancy is the biofeedback we yearn for. It's what fills our first chakra cup and teaches our nervous system how to move between agitation and calm. The safer we feel, the stronger our first chakra energy.

At a first chakra consciousness level, we also encode our tribe's beliefs as our rules, their fears as our dangers, and their treatment of us as a reflection of who we are and what we intrinsically deserve. It is as though we forever internalize our caregivers inside our first chakra, where they can keep reminding us of "the way things are."

As we grow, if our parents actively keep us safe and attend to our fears, we get the message that we are important and worthy of being cared for. We grow up with a built-in and regularly reinforced reality that *of course we matter*! By watching our parents intervene for us, advocate for us, actively keep us safe and happy, we learn that we have the right to be safe and supported no matter what. We also learn that not feeling safe is wrong and should be remedied.

Our first chakra develops mirroring this consciousness of well-being as the way things should be. We feel intrinsically safe because we belong and are loved and supported by a tribe that has our back. It won't occur to us to question whether we have the right to take up space, be who we are, and have the things we want. We matter.

Kids who grow up getting basic needs met and knowing without a doubt that they matter will stand up for themselves when something feels unfair. They feel grounded in their body and solid in their self-value. They carry a sense of well-being, lightness, and tolerance of modern-day risks such as making mistakes. They feel that the world in general is safe, and when life does get scary, they more easily reach out for the solid supportive tribe who will be there for them. Think of the child who, just before running into the playground, looks back to his mother for reassurance. When she returns his gaze with a warm, encouraging look of *It's okay and I am right here watching*, he's free to run into the unknown with abandon.

A strong Root Chakra in adulthood means the world is our oyster. We're confident enough to apply for that dream job, ask for more money, start a business, or just be ourselves. We can be highly creative and have fun while still being focused, practical, and balanced. We are bold, enthusiastic, and willing to risk the unknown. When we fail (as we all do), we know we will get over it because we have before. Because we expect to be supported, we easily ask for help when we need it. We are resilient when we venture off on our own, as if our first chakra has within it our solid support team standing with us, holding us, telling us it will be okay, and cheering us on—our tribe.

A FOUNDATION OF FEAR

If our first chakra cup has not been filled enough—if we generally don't feel safe and valued—our first chakra is more like an empty space where anxiety swirls and floats. With nothing to hold on to, fear, anxiety, panic, failure, and disappointment are ours to deal with alone. Where we're meant to feel solid inside feels shaky instead because it's built on a foundation of fear. This is not the healthy fear that alerts us to real danger and spurs us to respond but a gnawing feeling that somehow we just aren't safe, even during times when all is well.

Without an inner solid ground, anxiety can feel like falling backward into a terrifying nothingness, a black hole, and it is rarely soothed. We either don't go into the playground at all or we go but do our best not to be noticed. We're much more comfortable being invisible.

When *not* being lovingly attended to as a child is a daily consistent reality, the built-in messages are cemented into our chakra consciousness and nervous system. These are the deep roots of our beliefs that we are not important enough to be noticed, kept safe, reassured, and soothed. For some it's much worse. Abusive childhoods put the nervous system on high alert. We are always bracing for danger, as if we were in a war zone. Our first chakra is built around a devastating series of painful experiences that have taught us which actions or desires will be ignored, criticized, attacked, and punished. This becomes the seed of unworthiness that can underlie a lifetime of struggle.

This foundation of fear creates a lifelong hidden agenda: We will do whatever it takes to avoid feeling that awful space of inner anxiousness. Most of our actions, achievements, and ways of relating to others will center on trying to avoid feeling unsafe no matter what the cost. On the surface this can look like procrastination that seems frustratingly illogical but is secretly playing a key role in avoiding risk. Or we will work hard and overachieve to prove we are good enough to chase feeling safe, while inside always doubting our worth.

With a weak first chakra, we aren't fully present and grounded in our bodies but instead have excess energy up in our heads—racing, spinning, worrying, and overthinking. That frenetic energy leaves us with less energy down in our body, and other chakras suffer. Instead of our true brilliance, deeply felt passions, and wise heart guiding our actions, our mind and nervous system, wired for anxiety and derailed with safety and survival fears, are running the show.

UNQUESTIONED TRUTHS

Our early experiences of safety and survival form the foundational set point of how calm or anxious we feel in our body *as a way being.* They are also the beginning of what we understand to be true about ourselves, shaping our beliefs about our intrinsic worthiness and what we feel we have the right to ask for and expect. Our consistent experiences become the *unquestioned truths* we carry with us throughout life, and they are very powerful, forever influencing how we show up in the world.

People are surprised when they take stock of how many of their actions—including pursuits, successes, and mistakes—are driven in large part by trying to finally feel safe and belong.

Early Root Chakra programming affects the following:

- Whether our nervous system gets wired to feel generally safe or anxious
- How we experience our basic worthiness and right to be who we are
- How we feel about, notice, and take care of our physical body's needs
- Whether we easily get overstimulated and stressed out and how sensitive we are to our environments
- How much stress and anxiety we carry daily as we go about life

How do we carry the unquestioned truths we garnered as an infant and young child into adulthood? They get hardwired into our nervous system.

The Cost of a Weak First Chakra

- Difficulty getting into action
- Frenetic thoughts
- Anxious energy from mild to full-blown panic attacks
- Rejection of or disappointment in your physical body
- Difficulty being aware of your body's signals of stress, hunger, exhaustion
- "Leaving" your body and zoning out
- Dreaming of big goals that never manifest

- Difficulty creating the time or habit for nutrition and self-care
- Difficulty dealing with concrete tasks such as money management, organization, or finishing projects

Benefits of a Strong First Chakra

- Quantum leap in feeling grounded, safe, and powerfully embodied at the physical nervous-system level
- Experiencing the centered oneness and energy of deep self-love and acceptance of your physical body
- Feeling at ease in your body and being able to truly let go and relax (not be stuck in your head)
- Feeling the actual energy in your body of physical manifestation and magnetic attraction, heart energy, and embodied core energy that brings action
- Exuding a presence, energy, and "glow" that is noticeable and unforgettable to other people
- Being able to consciously catch, identify, and address habitual thoughts based on family paradigms and your first-chakra belief system so you can shift into the new reality you are creating

FEAR AND THE STRESS RESPONSE

Most of us have heard about the fight-or-flight response—also known as the stress response. The nervous system is naturally wired to sense and respond to fear and pain, and it's a pretty important aspect of what's known as the primitive, or reptilian, part of the brain. When faced with a stressor or frightening foe, stress hormones (adrenaline, noradrenaline, and cortisol) start pumping into our muscles, mobilizing us to act. Our heart pounds and rate of breathing accelerates. Designed to keep us alive in truly scary situations, the stress response gives the body enough of a jolt to effectively respond to real danger.

Responding appropriately to fear and pain can save our lives. When we're scared, we're given the strength to fight an enemy or run away—fast. If we are powerless to do either or shocked with fear, we might freeze instead, as if our conscious mind had left our body. As a survival mechanism, the freeze response is a way to stay unnoticed so our enemy, say an animal whose sight best detects motion, won't see us—or at least won't see us as a threat.

The fight-flight-freeze stress response seldom helps us in modern-day situations, where the dangers are more often about psychological or emotional pain than physical attack. The stress response is meant for short periods of real danger—in kill-or-be-killed situations. It was never intended to stay "on" during every-day life, yet many of us live in a state of chronic stress and anxiety because our weakened Root Chakra has been overwhelmed by external stressors. This state is incredibly taxing on the body and has a massive negative impact on our health and ability to think clearly and act decisively.

With a strong, intact Root Chakra, our nervous system is more resilient and less reactive. We trigger the stress response less often and are able to turn it off when the danger is gone. Our mind-body systems easily and regularly return to a relaxed rest-and-digest state. In this state our mind becomes calmer and more centered, and our thinking is clearer, inspired, and creative.

THE NERVOUS SYSTEM REMEMBERS

A weak first chakra means our nervous system is always on guard. Throughout life our nervous system will always remind us when it associates a particular situation or action as being unsafe by triggering the stress response automatically—even if we are only thinking about or imagining things from the past or future! This is great when we're in real danger. But when learned first-chakra fears get triggered, we're stressed out for no logical reason—and we have no control over this built-in primal mechanism. This is why willpower and logic are so ineffective in turning off anxiety about things such as public speaking, flying, elevators, and bugs, for instance.

Compounding matters is that the nervous system doesn't know the difference between true and false or past and present. It only knows the "charge" of past experiences that were shocking, painful, or dangerous and alerts us when anything that feels similar is happening again.

So, what happens when the childhood experiences we absorbed when our Root Chakra was developing lead us to believe something about ourselves or the world that isn't true? What happens when our perceptions, for whatever reason, are off base or distorted? What if many of our unquestioned truths about ourselves, what we deserve, and other people are completely false, as if we were looking in a faulty, fun-house mirror? We walk around feeling unsafe and on guard for no real reason.

Without a key to unlock these hardwired first-chakra associations about what is safe and not safe, we're basically at the mercy of our nervous system. Although we will have long forgotten about the beliefs and experiences that are driving these automatic reactions, the nervous system remembers.

Healing and rebuilding the Root Chakra starts with finding the source of these false fears and beliefs and letting them go. We must recognize when our nervous system is responding to what it considers to be a threat to survival based on how it's been wired at the Root Chakra level.

"BUT I HAD A GOOD CHILDHOOD!"

Life did not have to be demonstrably unsafe for us to carry excess anxiety or want to hide in the shadows instead of risking failure or criticism. The completely unguarded nervous system of an infant can absorb unintended traumas such as spending the first weeks of life with very little loving touch in the sterile environment of an incubator.

Loving parents who carry a lot of anxiety themselves sometimes aren't able to bring the calm energy needed to soothe a child. I have met many clients whose loving parents endured some tragedy, such as serious illness or the loss of a child, and were just unable to be fully attentive and present with them as children.

No one's childhood is perfect, and any stressful period in a family's life can create varying degrees of underlying feelings of unsafety and anxiousness. Financial strain, family strife, illness, and unemployment are some of the more subtle culprits. More obvious are growing up in a war zone or living through a natural disaster. Even watching these stressful situations on the news can elevate parental anxiety.

Many clients insist they had safe, loving childhoods and are unsure of the source of their constant need to stay busy and in control as a way to keep anxiety at bay. It often turns out that as soon as they were four or five, they picked up a different kind of unsafe feeling. For some, one or both parents were not sufficiently responsible or in charge. These kids learned early that they had to become the "parentified child" who puts childlike needs and fun aside to be the sacrificing caregiver.

Finally, many of my clients learned over time that it was more important to achieve than to be a child. Being a straight-A student, the best athlete on the team, or a perfectly behaved child was the standard. Anything less than perfect was ignored, criticized, or "a disappointment."

In all these cases, we will find it very hard to let go, ask others for support, or roll with our mistakes. Even trying to take our foot off the gas pedal can trigger anxiety because we're letting our guard down. "It's not worth it," we'll say, because it is just easier to always be in control and in motion.

UNSPOKEN AND PREVERBAL TRIBAL RULES: SURVIVAL = BELONGING = BONDING

As we grow, the Root Chakra grows and develops with us, and our collection of unquestioned truths expands. Even as toddlers we start to take in more sophisticated information and unquestioned truths from our parents, as feeling safe takes on a new social dimension: belonging.

A primitive survival reality is that doing something that upsets our tribe can lead to judgment, rejection, and consequently being outcast—a sure threat to survival. The best way to ensure we belong and are therefore safe within our tribe is to figure out and follow the rules, which often means acting agreeable and accommodating while forgoing our unique desires.

Because our parents are in charge, their rules and norms are of utmost importance. We quickly take note of them, even at the tender age of toddlerhood. The actual rules as well as the way we learn them matter to our developing Root Chakra. Do the rules teach us how to be happy and successful and expand at each stage of development, or do they damage our growing sense of self and empowerment? Are we learning them through consistent directions, reminders, and thoughtful consequences or through consistent fear, shame, and punishments? This process is the next critical piece of how we experience the Root Chakra.

As we become more and more developmentally independent, the second chakra energy of needs, wants, and impulses starts to emerge. How our tribe reacts to these natural desires impacts us at the first chakra—and this is when life starts to get complicated! We can't wait to express ourselves, but, inevitably, our tribe is not excited about everything we feel compelled to do. Some of our new actions are encouraged and applauded—such as when we're good to a younger sibling. But some actions are met with displeasure, and that's how we know we have broken a rule.

We don't judge the norms but accept them, even if they are painful, random, or unhealthy. Our survival depends upon it. We viscerally (not logically) expect some sort of punishment if we break a rule—rejection, criticism, attack, abandonment—and the sinking feeling that goes with it.

Year by year, as we continue to figure out and experience our family's rules and punishments, we learn how to survive them instead of how to thrive in life. We will adapt by acting meek, scared, or small to exude the *I know I am not good enough or special* demeanor that will preempt attack and keep the peace. We will shame ourselves out of doing something before our caregivers have a chance to do so and therefore we don't arouse the scariest and most shocking type of retribution—shaming and/or physical attack.

The "bond to survive in the tribe" response is really the root of shame, or the notion that we (not what we did but our innate impulses) are bad. As we get older and our other chakras start to develop, we will feel shame or guilt whenever we feel compelled to follow a previously shamed impulse—to do something that will have the tribe acting aghast or angry.

We'll talk more about shame in Chapter 5, but it's important to see shame for what it really is: survival fear designed to stop us before we break family rules that are contrary to our natural, built-in human needs, desires, and wants. Being shamed always turns into self-shame. It invites us not to follow through with our natural desires, which are meant to drive us in the direction of our expansion, growth, dreams, and ultimately our life's purpose. Fear, anxiety, shame, and the survival instinct, now firmly embedded in our first-chakra foundation, move with us into adulthood, affecting every aspect of how we function in life.

EARNING THE RIGHT TO FEEL SAFE: HIGH ACHIEVERS, PERFECTIONISM, AND SELF-DOUBT

In adulthood self-shame as a survival mechanism evolves into smart-sounding self-doubt. Many driven and successful super-achievers will say they don't think they struggle with fear or anxiety and certainly not the low self-esteem of shame. However, if they drop a ball or don't know how to do something right the first time or make a mistake—if they are exposed in any way—they admit to being overcome with massive amounts of anxiety. The first-chakra fear equating failure or imperfection with life-or-death unsafety takes over. These folks have a solid enough first chakra to be successful in business but must always *earn their right to feel safe* by vigilantly following the rules of being perfect or successful.

As adults high achievers have to adapt how they earn the right to feel safe. They are constantly working, doing, exercising, and achieving, balancing ten things at once so they never have to feel that anxiety. Feeling anxiety is confusing to them because they are so successful in some ways—they're not frozen and hiding at home. But in other ways, they are plagued with self-doubt. They feel incredibly insecure, one mistake away from being judged a failure or a fraud. One mistake away from being overcome with shame.

In successful circles self-shame is associated with unworthiness and low self-esteem, neither of which fits the identity of a high achiever. However, self-doubt can live loud and large in our head as a "frenemy," seemingly pushing us to try harder, make sure everything is right, and do better next time by smartly reminding us of all of our failures.

For example, high-achieving professional women may want nothing more than to climb the ladder. But when increasingly under the spotlight, they can be overwhelmed and paralyzed with a sudden onslaught of self-doubt. This can be infuriating, as they don't understand why they can't step up with confidence, own their value, or market themselves boldly. This is the conundrum of procrastinating when we consciously really want and need to act.

It takes a great deal of time to convince 90 percent of my clients that fear is at the root of why they procrastinate instead of show up, spin with self-doubt instead of take action, or overwork themselves instead of set boundaries. Most of them have been racking their brains to figure out why they behave this way and to find the next magic-bullet strategy. But we can't trust the mind when it comes to this. It's directly related to the nervous system's fight-flight-freeze-*bond* wiring, or how we've been conditioned to respond automatically to a threat to our safety—our survival.

TRIBALISM BEYOND FAMILY

When it comes to the first chakra, family is our first tribe but not our last. All groups and institutions are tribe-like, with spoken and unspoken rules, norms, and consequences. The bond response is a common automatic survival tool that can baffle and disempower us in any modern-day tribal setting. To ensure we are always in the protective bubble of belonging, our instinct can make us act agreeable and accommodating at the expense of our unique desires. Our bonding behavior is not based on true shared interests or beliefs but is an automatic self-censorship done out of fear. We don't want to rock the boat.

As adults in the workplace, for instance, we step into many new tribes—co-workers, management, the boardroom, clients—and unconsciously carry with us our deeply rooted childhood life-or-death rules. Some of these new tribes reinforce those rules. Reacting negatively to confidence and assertiveness is a big one. Other tribes are overtly abusive, conveying the message that *You don't matter, you are powerless, and if you say anything, you will be punished/fired.* The specter of being punished becomes the adult fear of being fired, which, of course, is a legitimate survival fear!

In the workplace people can be physically, emotionally, sexually, and verbally abused. Or they might be systematically undervalued and underpaid as part of a long-standing culture of discrimination based on gender, race, religion, or sexual orientation. This picture has been painted many times over in other settings as well.

The many Me Too revelations, even in trusted organizations, including the church, emphasize the power of the tribe and the will to bond. These traumatizing sexual abuse events have not only damaged people's lives but left the survivors to wonder why they froze, did not speak up, and "let it happen." They look back with confusion about why they submitted, played along, or apologized and made excuses for bad actors when they were so egregiously being wronged. What looks so clear in retrospect makes it all the harder for them to understand how they acted. Time and time again, they ask themselves, *Why didn't I have the courage or presence of mind to stand up for myself?* They blame themselves and, heartbreakingly, fear being blamed by others.

If only they understood the overriding power of a tribe to trigger first-chakra survival fear—activating the nervous system and kicking us into automatic reactions. This is what makes us freeze and resort to the bonding behaviors of shrinking down, giving in, laughing along, or even acting compassionate and understanding. If only they understood that at that moment, they had no presence of mind because their mind, outrage, and courage were being hijacked by deeply entrenched tribal fears and survival behaviors.

My driving passion and fury is to help those who have been wronged and then silenced to finally understand this dynamic so they can give themselves (and ask for) the love and compassion they truly deserve as someone who was wronged and traumatized. The Heart Chakra chapter will address this specifically as a continuation of our healing journey in this book.

HEALING THE FIRST CHAKRA

Of all the chakras, the Root Chakra is the one we're most unaware of, which is why I believe it is typically the least explored in personal growth. It's highly connected to our primitive survival adaptations—fight, flight, freeze, or bond—and involves delving into and tolerating uncomfortable feelings. These feelings produce the illogical life-or-death sweat responses that do not serve us.

It's hard to imagine that our fear of public speaking is linked to a *Don't act like you're so special* rule that got secretly coded into our nervous system 20, 40, or 60 years ago. It's even harder to accept that it's wired into the part of the brain responsible for our survival. Public speaking, for instance, is generally a safe proposition. It won't kill us. Yet that's how it can feel to anyone who learned early in life that it is safer to stay in your lane, and your lane is *Don't look too confident—or else.*

A good way to understand how your first chakra is filled is by imagining that your parents or other significant tribe members (as they looked when you were growing up) are standing inside your first chakra, actively reacting to everything you are doing. Much like the child who looks back to a parent for support, encouragement, assurance, safety, and unconditional love when unsure or in need of soothing, you check in with them for their reaction.

All of us need to heal and rebuild the first chakra to some degree. Tapping is the perfect modality for addressing first-chakra pain because it's a direct line to the nervous system, capable of swiftly turning off the stress response when it comes to anxiety and shame. We can effectively dull the impact of childhood traumas, soothe our anxiety, and turn down the power and volume of childhood rules and unquestioned truths, even those that started in utero. We can reduce or eliminate ungrounding fearful thinking, own our presence, and set a powerful foundation upon which our other chakras can rely.

Healing usually produces an unexpected byproduct: Miraculously, unsupportive people from our first-chakra-internalized tribe not only lose their hold on us but either change for the better or are no longer prominent figures in our lives. This usually opens up an opportunity to intentionally add new tribal members—people of our own choosing.

As adults we can consciously choose a new group of trusted people who are there for us, have our back, encourage us, and act as our safety net—people we know will reinforce our worth, gifts, and courage while accepting us for our fears, insecurities, and flaws. As we form a new tribe with people we trust, they become the people standing in our first chakra whom we can look back to for our internal check-in.

COMMENTARY BY DAVID RANIERE, PH.D.

We need to know where we come from. Ultimately, there is incredible power in such knowing. Our ability to plant our feet firmly on the ground and stand strong, claim a life for ourselves that fully expresses who we are, and recover from those moments when we are completely thrown off balance depends on having a solid foundation.

Some of us are fortunate to have had that solid foundation from the beginning and are quite proud of our roots, whereas others carry burdens and scars of deep and abiding shame, doubt, fear, and inhibition. These are the sorrowful legacies of a painful childhood. All of us—whether we identify with either, neither, or some blend of these two groups—carry into our adult lives a complex imprint that is unique to our distinct life story. I have never met anyone for whom this has not been true.

Our roots are where our layered lives began. I say "layered" because there are (at least) three interconnected realms of human experience in which we are rooted. On the concrete (physiological) level, our body self is rooted in constitutional predispositions, such as our temperament, and includes aspects of our wiring and genetic code that shape the expression of our physical selves. These ingredients or building materials were not of our own choosing but nonetheless exert an enormous influence in shaping our sense of who we are.

On the interpersonal (relationship) level, our earliest roots are anchored in our primary attachment bonds. These are the bonds we formed with the most important of relationships—our parents and early caregivers on whom our very lives depended.

And on the intrapsychic (mental/psychological) level, our mind creates from patterns of interaction with others and the outside world a set of organizing blueprints (sometimes referred to as internal working models) that direct our attention and inform how we perceive and understand ourselves and our environment.

To grasp how important and formative our early experiences are—and how they shape who we think we are (and just as importantly, who we think we're not)—we need to keep all three of these realms in mind as we reach back to a time before we can remember.

Reaching this far back into our personal history feels like a stretch because it is, and the idea of it awakens the skeptic in many of us. It is important to strive to remain grounded solidly in truth whenever we construct a story about forces that have shaped who we are. At the same time, however, our earliest life experiences—from being in the womb through infancy and the first several years of early childhood—are chapters of our lives that cannot be remembered in the conventional sense no matter how hard we try. The vast majority of what happened then was encoded in our nervous system and cannot be "fact-checked"; consequently, we can assert only a limited set of claims about "what really happened" back then.

This inherent limitation is something we cannot overcome because it derives from an inescapable truth about brain development: Our brains need to develop enough to be capable of various cognitive abilities. For example, the ability to use language to represent experience and communicate takes time to develop (and one of the joys of parenthood is having front-row seats, watching in awe as this process unfolds in the developing child). Similarly, the brain's memory center, especially the hippocampus, takes time to develop.

We cannot simply recall events from early childhood because our brains were not developed enough to encode and store our experience in memory. As a result, when we try to retrieve information about our earliest experiences directly, we are inevitably at a loss.

So how are we to make contact with early-childhood experiences given this limitation? First we need to keep in mind that even though we did not encode experiences in memory like we do now, we absorbed everything. Our body's developing nervous system took it all in and, like a sponge, absorbed the countless sensory experiences from inside and outside to which it was exposed.

One of the world's foremost experts on trauma, Bessel van der Kolk, M.D., has put it plainly in his seminal work by the same title: "The body keeps the score." Our bodies remember. And one of the ways we have access to how the body remembers is through what we feel.

Please take a moment here to pause and really take that in. Here's another pass at it: *the body tells us what it remembers through what we feel.*

This simple principle is an extremely powerful one that I draw upon in both my clinical work and my personal life in ways that extend far beyond matters we typically think of as involving trauma. For example, whenever I am sitting with a patient who is feeling anxious or afraid of something that might happen, I relate to their experience in two ways. I listen first to exactly what they are saying about what they are scared of, and I attend to it as a completely real and legitimate concern. At the same time, I am also hearing what they are saying as a statement about something that has already happened.

As you read this, you may be saying to yourself, *Wait a second! How could something that hasn't happened yet have happened already?* But before you put the book down, take a moment to consider the possibility that if you are scared of something happening, it already has.

To be afraid of something, we must already know that there is something to be afraid of, even if we aren't consciously thinking about anything in particular from the past or don't have any memory of an experience that might be relevant to the present or future concern. In the simplest of terms, this is how the body keeps the score, or how our nervous system holds within it a history we don't even remember and remains poised to make us aware of it again by representing it to us as a feeling state.

If we begin to relate to what we are feeling now in this way, something profound happens. Our relationship to our internal experience expands as we are no longer limited to thinking in linear, concrete, and rational or logical terms. Our field of consciousness opens up to include where we are rooted in our nervous system. Instead of only locating something as ahead of us that we are bracing for, we begin to consider that something may be coming in from "the beyond"—from a past we cannot remember that is presencing (i.e., re-present-ing) itself in the feeling we are having.

The feeling *is* the memory—a memory without words, a visual image, or the narrative structure of a remembered story. In the moment, a strong emotion can feel like a lightning bolt striking down on us from the sky. In fact it is a charge rising up from the ground—a charge rooted in a nervous-system activation—that is rising up to the body's surface.

Margaret's guided tapping and visualization processes are designed to invite this nervous-system activation. The idea is to reach back into the beyond and bring into the present that which is there but may not be remembered, something akin to what the psychoanalyst Christopher Bollas (1987) calls the "unthought known."

But before we get there, there is something else we can do to address the question I posed earlier about the challenge of making contact with early-childhood experience given the constraints imposed by the developmental process itself. We can also draw upon the study of human development as a guide and make informed inferences based on rigorous empirical research. We can hold those findings up against the light of our personal sensibility and see if it fits.

Yes, we bring normative data to our felt sense of our experience and use our best judgment. A useful guide as we do this is to notice what our bodies tell us as we read this book and participate in the guided processes. I encourage you to have in the back of your mind questions such as: *Is this resonating with me? Does my response to this process bring up a feeling, a thought, a memory from another time in my life, or an image that offers confirmation or disconfirmation of its validity?*

The Still-Face Effect: Developmental Research and the First Chakra

During the 1975 meeting of the Society for Research in Child Development, psychologist Edward Tronick, Ph.D., and his colleagues first presented their findings on the Still-Face Experiment, which today remains one of the most replicated research findings in developmental psychology (Tronick, Als, and Adamson 1978; Adamson and Frick 2003; Mesman, van IJzendoorn, and Bakermans-Kranenburg 2009).[1]

In this powerful experiment, a mother (or other primary caregiver) and infant (ranging in age from 1 to 12 months) are filmed while they sit a few feet apart from each other in a video laboratory. The mother and infant's natural interactions are observed. Typically, a lovely exchange familiar to us all then unfolds. The mother takes the lead in engaging the baby and his current emotional state, matching facial expressions and vocal tones as the pair begins to synchronize in a shared experience of the moment, locking into each other's gaze. Within 30 seconds they are having the time of their lives, cooing and cawing, smiling and taking each other in as they connect playfully in this improvisational dance. Then the mother is instructed via an earpiece to "go still." She is to simply wipe any expression from her face, assume a neutral gaze, and sit still in front of her baby.

The profound change that consistently occurs in the infant in response to the mother's still face is the most important (and

1 Dr. Tronick is director of the Infant-Parent Mental Health program at the University of Massachusetts Boston, where he conducts research on maternal depression and other stressors that affect the emotional development and health of infants and children. His work overlaps with that of the Boston Change Process Study Group, a group of psychoanalysts and developmentalists who study infant and child development and its application to the psychotherapeutic change process.

very-upsetting-to-watch) part of this experiment. Immediately aware of this abrupt change, the baby first stares back at the mother as if looking for her. He then offers a brief smile or some other behavioral bid to reengage and revive the shared state they were in just moments ago. When the mother's nonresponsiveness continues, the baby turns away only to look back at her again, periodically monitoring her state and repeating this cycle of attempting to solicit his mother's attention.

Within the next couple of minutes, the baby becomes increasingly distressed as these efforts fail repeatedly, and his efforts to reestablish connection with his mother grow increasingly desperate. Vocalizations become high-pitched screeches and screams, he thrusts his entire body toward the mother with outstretched arms, and his entire muscular system becomes rigid with tension. All efforts at self-soothing then fail, and this gives way to a loss of postural control and the infant literally droops down and slumps over. Accompanying this physical collapse, the baby's face flushes red, his gaze is cast down and to the right, and he enters a profoundly disengaged state of withdrawal and remains there until his mother is instructed to emerge from the still-face condition.

Important inferences about infants' experiences during the still-face experiment have been drawn, and prominent theories have been advanced based on these inferences (for a review, see Adamson and Frick, 2003). For our purposes, I want to anchor us in a couple of core ideas related to the first chakra and the nervous system assaults that are encoded in the body at the first chakra level.

First the study powerfully demonstrates the reality of social interaction and social embeddedness that exists at the very beginning of life. We all exist as part of a larger social unit—what Margaret refers to as a tribe—from the start. The smallest and most important tribal unit with which we are embedded and have the most direct contact is the parent-child dyad.

For the infant and developing child, the other person with whom we connect becomes the first mirror in which we see ourselves. What is reflected (and not reflected) back to us from that other person has a profound impact on our physical and emotional experience of ourselves. Tronick and colleagues (1998) refer to this as "dyadic states of consciousness," the shared states inhabited by both mother and infant when they are engaged in an interconnected (i.e., intersubjective) experience of meaningful interaction.

The still-face moment represents a break in this vital connected state, and what we see in the infant is a profoundly distressing nervous system assault involving a spiraling out of a relationship and into a painfully withdrawn state of aloneness.

Along with underscoring the fact of our embeddedness within a relationship, the still-face effect also draws attention to the importance of what is shared within that dyad. The mother's still face represents one form of sudden withdrawal and nonengagement. But there are many other forms of an almost still face, when the face looking back at the infant isn't exactly still but may be depressed or somewhat withdrawn, anxious or intrusive, absent or preoccupied, or disparaging or critical. These kinds of reflections back to the infant are encoded into its implicit experience of relating, as part of the shared consciousness we invisibly inhabit long before there are words or thoughts to separate ourselves from them.

Remember Margaret's story of the old, damaged fun-house mirror at the start of the Introduction? That kind of mirror is often rooted in patterned exchanges in which what was reflected back to us in the eyes of a parent left us seeing ourselves in some warped or distorted way.

I will address the vital role of affect in Chapter 13, when we discuss the Heart Chakra, but as Margaret points out in this chapter, the roots of shame begin at the first chakra. From the beginning of life, infants are keyed into their parents' shifting states and register changes in them that are far less dramatic than a still face. To stay alive and continue to feel ourselves in relationships with those who keep us alive, as babies and children, we adjust accordingly to the states of those around us without even thinking about it. This simple form of nonverbal learning is what all animals figure out: *When I do this, that happens; when I don't do this, something else happens.* It's when we first begin to learn who to be and who not to be in order to keep other people around so we can get our basic needs met enough to survive.

The still-face experiments give us insight about a time before we had words or thoughts for our experiences, to the realm of the beyond that predates cognitive memory. In fact one of the most compelling formulations of the still-face effect is that it is the earliest form of what becomes the emotional state we call shame.

I will elaborate on this further when we return to the discussion of shame at the second chakra level, but for now I want to emphasize the direct nervous system (parent) to nervous system (infant) contact that is made at the first charka level during early life and how that is absorbed into the being of the developing child. We experienced these states during a time before we could tell time—one that we cannot remember directly and for which there weren't words. And it is here that tapping offers us hope as a vehicle to access that realm. Engaging the nervous system directly provides us a method by which we can make contact with and ultimately bring comfort and calm to what remains held in the body.

CHAPTER 2

HEALING YOUR FRIGHTENED INNER CHILD

This chapter introduces the first of three guided Healing Experiences for the Root Chakra. The goal here sounds pretty lofty: we're going to enroll your younger self (your inner child) to help transform your first chakra. Using visualization, we're going back in time to uncover and heal the root cause of your earliest nervous system wiring around fear, anxiety, safety, and feelings of being unwanted. It's not as daunting as it sounds—and it's incredibly effective.

No one consciously remembers their birth, although you may have some adult knowledge of events or what your parents were dealing with at the time. Without remembering your birth, you're going to set an intention to see what your young and immature nervous system sensed about feeling safe, soothed, and taken care of as a newborn. These are critical first experiences that become wired into your nervous system and set the foundation for your first chakra development.

As you work with the exercises in this chapter, recognize that there is a vast range of human experience, from abuse and neglect to sensing something was "off" to complete love, attention, and care. The scripts are geared to voice emotionally intense feelings.

If it feels extreme to you, that's okay. There's no harm in reciting the script while you're tapping.

If you visualize a warm, loving picture, be happy that you may not need to do much work in this first exercise. If that's the case, I encourage you to be curious and look deeper to find something else that might present itself. For example, you may see a safe, loved infant, and then your unconscious may suddenly fast-forward to a moment in kindergarten when you felt scared and alone. This is the intrinsic intelligence of the mind-body system offering you something that does need healing and compassion. Alternatively, you can skip to the final tapping script and visualization (#1-3) in this chapter—healing the inner child—to surround the image of your younger self with even more unconditional love.

For some of you, this process may be emotionally intense, but know that tapping will keep moving your nervous system through the wave from triggered to calm. You will progress to the point where you feel lighter and relieved.

HEALING EXPERIENCE #1: HEALING YOUR FRIGHTENED INNER CHILD

Setup Visualization #1-1

To get started sit in a quiet, comfortable place in an upright position with your feet on the floor. Close your eyes and take a series of deep belly breaths. For a few seconds, feel down into your feet. Try to feel the bottoms of your feet where they are touching the floor. Then feel into the chair or couch you are sitting on, noticing everywhere your body is making contact and being supported, from your legs to behind to your back. This quick process, which you will use throughout the Healing Experiences, will help to put you in a light meditative state.

Next, visualize that you are looking at a movie screen in your mind's eye, where your unconscious mind can easily paint a picture or show a movie clip. You can even set a conscious intention out loud, requesting permission from your unconscious mind to do this easily.

Now let your unconscious mind paint a picture of a tiny baby that is clearly you. Maybe you were just born, or maybe you're a couple of weeks old. Be curious about that. It's okay if it feels as if you're making something up or remembering an old photograph. Trust that your mind will paint the picture that you need to see.

See that baby there and just breathe. Now look for and allow more details to materialize as the picture becomes more of a movie clip. Notice whether it's daytime or nighttime and where the baby is—inside, outside, in the hospital? Is the baby alone or is someone nearby? Get those impressions. There are no right or wrong answers. We're not looking for a specific memory. The intention is to see what needs to be healed. It is more about allowing a picture to appear and trusting that what appears is important to explore.

Notice how your mind is painting the picture or giving you impressions by taking in how the baby looks. Is the little one happy and safe or crying and alone? Because we are looking with the intention of healing feelings of unsafety, imagine you could check in with the baby about how true the following statement is on a scale of 0 to 10, where 0 is not true at all and 10 is completely true: "I don't feel safe, something is wrong, and I am afraid."

If you feel completely safe (1), I invite you to bless that happy moment! As mentioned above, you can skip to the tapping script and visualization #1-3 and surround the baby with love, or you can see whether your unconscious wants to present another image for when you didn't feel safe.

Another variation to use when everything feels safe is to bring in the conscious awareness of a big goal, if you have one. Most big goals represent going beyond our parents' limits or experiences. Consider how your goal, when accomplished, represents how you want to be standing in your power. Are you earning well, being rewarded, and enjoying life? Many I have worked with have found it powerful to see how holding a big goal for the future impacts this exercise because it may represent no longer fitting in with your family.

I have done this exercise with thousands of people from all over the world and draw on that here and throughout the book for the tapping phrases. These phrases are based on the check-in sentence "I don't feel safe" feeling very true.

Now it's time to jump in and start tapping through the points. For a refresher on how to tap, revisit the Tapping section in the Introduction.

Tapping Script #1-1

There I am, just this small one – I just came through into this tiny body, into this tiny nervous system – And I'm flooded with physical feelings and sensations – And it's scary – My nervous system is overwhelmed with sensations – Maybe at times safe and loved – Warm and fed – And at other times alone – Maybe even screaming, sad, alone – And the question within me – Am I meant to be here? – Do these people really want me? – Because they're not soothing me – Somehow I don't feel safe – They are not making me feel safe – Did I come to the wrong family?

There I am crying, screaming, angry, scared – Maybe I had trauma at birth – Something shocking and scary happened – Maybe I was isolated when I needed to be held and soothed, or maybe I learned right away – That I wasn't wanted – Maybe I felt immediately something was off – That I wasn't fully wanted – Or maybe not wanted at all – Maybe I sensed that even in loving me – My parents were limited – Maybe stressed, anxious, conflicted – Maybe there were parts of me they wouldn't want to see.

There I am, this tiny child – Fear gripping my nervous system – Maybe there is even shock and confusion – There I am, maybe feeling at times – Is this how it's going to be? – And with that is a terrible feeling – From this tiny state so vulnerable – I can't get away from this terrible feeling – There I am, my nervous system running with energy – My nervous system flooding with painful, unsoothed feelings – My nervous system running with energy – I totally honor this baby – I totally honor my first chakra.

Take a deep breath.

If your picture resonated with the words in the script, your emotions were likely intense. If so, it is best to repeat the round of tapping. Either way take a moment to just be with the gravity of what your unconscious revealed to you. You may be seeing a representation of how your nervous system was wired long ago to always feel on alert and unsafe—how it was wired to find it difficult to relax into good feelings.

I Didn't Feel *Anything*

If your little one felt upset and unsafe, but during the tapping, you felt nothing, that's okay. It happens. Some of us have a finely tuned habit of protecting ourselves from feeling too much for fear it might overwhelm us. This self-protective strategy is usually quite effective as an emotional and psychological survival mechanism, and we want to respect it.

One approach is to consciously recognize and honor that inner resistance. Knowing you carry resistance is almost like a bonus—an additional aha moment about the amount of fear, hurt, and grief you are carrying. Be with that. You can then check in to see whether it's okay to give yourself permission to feel only a tiny fraction of what might be there—even if it is only one percent! If so, continue tapping. If not, you may want to seek support from a qualified and experienced tapping practitioner. That's okay too.

Setup Visualization #1-2

As we continue with this healing process, we want to check back in and see how the image has changed or shifted. So close your eyes and tune back into the baby and see how the baby looks now. Sometimes after the first round of tapping, you will have a clearer impression about what the baby is feeling. For some the baby may be more upset but with different emotions. Is it anger? Is it terror? Is it shock? Is it confusion? Is it like, *What am I doing here? This is wrong*? Really get clear on what it is.

If the baby looks less upset and calmer, look closely for more layers of feeling. The first round of tapping helps most people hold the space to lean in more fully to painful feelings so they can be voiced, honored, and released.

In this second round of tapping, we are now holding the space for the feelings of anger, hurt, and unfairness that can arise, especially if the words of fear in round one felt true. This script offers some phrases that will lead you to a full emotional release.

Tapping Script #1-2

There I am – It's really hard to see this – I don't really want to see this picture – The fear and aloneness and confusion – In such a tiny body – The aloneness and deprivation ripping through my system – Maybe even anger – Because at some level I knew – What I can see clearly now – It's not supposed to be this way – Maybe there was even a reaction of anger in my whole body – Maybe at my parents or even at God – An angry question – Why did you send me to these people? – This is a mistake – This is a mistake – I'm not supposed to be here – Too much pain – So much fear and agitation in my little nervous system – That must have felt like raw pain through my nervous system.

I'm just going to honor that – And these swirling questions – This confusion – From the earliest moments I had confusion – Why am I here? – This is wrong – This doesn't make sense – They're supposed to love me – They're supposed to keep me safe – And they're not – It's their one job to keep me safe – Anger mixed with fear in my tiny body – And I've carried it my whole life – Poor little me – Anger and fear in my nervous system – And I've carried it my whole life – Anger and fear that always comes first because of this.

Take a deep breath.

Many clients over the years have been astounded after that tapping round because they say that throughout their entire lives they have carried a feeling that they don't belong in their family or even here on the planet. Others see why they always feel unsafe and have a hard time sleeping or relaxing.

It is less important to know all the details about what happened or how your parents acted than it is to see the early seeds of beliefs being planted at a sensory level in your nervous system. Your unconscious mind may well be showing you in story form the raw feelings that have impacted your lifelong general sense of safety, well-being, and calm.

Tapping Script #1-3

There I am – Poor little me – I was just a baby – An innocent baby – Perfect – How could I not be perfect? – I can see the truth now – As a baby, I was, of course, lovable and deserving of love – I was always deserving of love and care – I deserved not only care but adoring attention – I needed and should have gotten soothing – Calming – Arms holding me with love – I didn't get what I needed – For all sorts of reasons that are less important now – But my nervous system has held on to this charged information –I always deserved that loving attention – There was nothing wrong with me – And I always deserved to be born – To be here – To be loved so much that I was soothed, held, and kept safe.

Maybe I have doubted that, but that was a mistake – I deserved unconditional love – And because I was helpless, I needed them to bring that to me – To give that to me – And though I may not have gotten that – I always deserved to be held in love – Surrounded by safe arms and soothed.

I am open to healing these raw emotional moments from my first chakra – Healing and releasing them from my nervous system – For my highest good – I deserve that – I am open to a new truth unfolding throughout my being – That I matter and have the right to feel safe, soothed, and loved – My fears and needs deserve to be heard and attended to – They always have – And I am open to attending to my own system – When I am anxious, overtired, overwhelmed, or hungry – I am open to taking care of myself with kindness – Because I deserve that.

Take a deep breath.

Post-Tapping Visualization #1-3

Take another deep breath. Tune into the baby again. Sometimes, even if the process wasn't intense for you, the picture suddenly looks different after you do more tapping. The baby will appear more at ease, and you will have the impression that the baby knows you are there watching, hearing, and validating them.

See that little one there, step in as the adult you are today, and bring love to that baby. Tell the baby, "It's okay. I'm here for you." This baby lives in your heart. This baby lives inside of you like an inner child, or more accurately, one of your inner-child selves. You can keep the little one safe now.

Let the baby know, "I'm going to be here for you. I'm going to keep you safe. It's okay." And tell the baby, "I understand. I understand. I am the only one who does."

Imagine that you could expand your Heart Chakra, and its beautiful spring-green color envelops you and the little child. Imagine that you could pour love from your heart into theirs. It's so easy to pour love toward the child. And if you're willing, love that little child even with their rage, because there's potential for every child to experience that emotion. Let them know you're loving them with their faults, their humanity, and with their body. You're loving them for their flaws as well as their gifts. You're loving them unconditionally—like an amazing aunt or uncle who swoops in to be there for that child when the child's parents can't be there.

Now tell the child something very important: "You have the right to be here. You have always deserved to be here. You have always deserved the unconditional love that brings soothing, calming, and safety. You belong here." And if you feel some resistance to that, it's okay. Just note it. You'll be working on it. And say to the child, "I have the right to be here, to be seen, to be accepted, and to be loved. I belong right here where I am."

And now shift the picture. Be in this present moment sitting in your chair wherever you are with your feet on the floor. Feel solid in your body. Let your mind come down into your body, feel your feet where they touch the floor. Feel the chair supporting you and your backside against the chair. Tune into the beautiful red energy of your grounded first chakra as if you are a solid oak tree with deep roots holding fast in the earth.

Imagine that you can surround yourself and the baby in that warm red energy and in the solid belief that *I belong here. I am safe, loved, and deserving. I am claiming my space and the energy of my first chakra.* Bring this red energy in and watch as the red glow turns to white and that little one melts right into your heart where they can always be safe and loved by *you* because you are the only one who truly understands and can bring the love and reassurance that they need.

Let the little one rest and be soothed and held in your heart, and notice how you feel in your body and in your heart. What are the feelings and sensations? What is different? Have you ever felt this way before? What did your unconscious reveal to you through this child? Write down or journal about any aha moments you have during these tapping sessions so you can sit with them later.

Again, it is less important to see historically accurate scenarios. These visualizations are more about finding and bringing your loving attention to early feelings of unsoothed unsafety or aloneness. Those intense moments can be running your nervous system in a pervasive, underlying way, as if it's reminding you every day that you are not safe in the world.

That's not true, but your nervous system reacts as if it were: *There is no safe, loving presence holding you, no one really cares, abandonment happens, and danger lurks around the corner—and you will always be alone in that.* This paradigm blocks the first chakra and zaps your energy. It is draining and exhausting, but it can be healed.

NEXT STEPS . . .

Over the next week or so, take a minute or two every day to sit and feel into your body. Put your hand on your heart and ask that little one what it needs. Listen, and then just be there with that for a few minutes. Then offer some words to this newly discovered inner child that they need or want to hear. This is the beginning of a new relationship of seeing, hearing, and lovingly attending to a long-ignored or avoided side of yourself—your anxious side, which is desperately seeking safety and love.

Visit www.unblockedbook.com/chapter2 for an extra tapping experience and discussion to enhance this chapter.

CHAPTER 3

HEALING THE BODY

We all know how important it is to take care of ourselves for health reasons. Few people, however, consider how essential it is to love and accept the body by treating it with compassion, kindness, and respect. Loving your body is important for many reasons.

To begin with, your body *is* your first chakra. It's the foundation of power upon which everything else in your energy system is built. It's the level of consciousness that represents all that is solid and tangible in your life. It's the means by which you manifest material things and circumstances into your life.

Second, being in your body—being present—is crucial to feeling alive and healthy and to being in action. When you're fully present, you are also better able to manifest. When you are not "in your body," you feel scattered and ungrounded, and you will seem scattered and ungrounded to other people as well. Your presence will not have much power or impact. Sometimes people will not even notice you.

Most of us don't love our bodies fully but reject aspects of them. Rejecting any part of your body is rejecting your first chakra and the empowerment energy it's meant to bring to you. Body rejection disconnects you from your physical self, which means you can't be fully present and so are not fully alive. Yet most people experience body rejection. They feel angry, disappointed, and even disgusted by their bodies.

Body rejection begins in different ways and at different times in life. As children maybe other kids insulted us or made us feel less than for being overweight, having a disability, or being unique or awkward in some way. A serious disease, illness, injury, or chronic pain can trigger anger, a lack of forgiveness, or grief and disappointment toward the body as well.

In this Healing Experience, you're going to look at how you feel about your physical body. You will have a mix of good and bad feelings, but this process can unearth some extremely unkind opinions about, and rejection of, your physical self. It can get intense! But to achieve a deep level of healing and bring you more into your most powerful presence, you need to look honestly at what you dislike about your body. I'm going to challenge you to look underneath some of your self-judgments and see the hurt, aloneness, and fear that is the true pain your body is carrying.

Healing body rejection has a major impact on your willingness to be in your body, or to be "embodied," and positively affects your energy and presence all around. It is also the key to increasing awareness of your body's signals about what you are feeling and needing. As a bonus your feelings and thoughts about your body will be more balanced, less distorted, and more loving.

Rebuilding the first chakra is noticing, hearing, and bringing love, soothing, and safety to spaces filled with old pain. It is not something you do once. It is a process of changing the habitual ways in which we reject and abandon ourselves. So expect to repeat this Healing Experience as needed.

HEALING EXPERIENCE #2: HEALING THE BODY

Setup Visualization #2-1

Start by taking a deep breath. Close your eyes and tune into your body. In that movie screen of your mind, picture a mirror in front of you. In that mirror you see your reflection, just as you are dressed today. Really notice and consider your body.

First, notice if there is something about your body that you really don't like and that you judge. Maybe it's not the way you want it to be, or it feels imperfect or not good enough in some way. Notice if you look at a part of you and say to yourself, *That is ugly.*

Second, let your mind run through the past and come up with a time when your body really let you down physically—a time when it disappointed you. Maybe you had an illness or an issue with something in your body that created pain, or your body didn't recover properly, or you needed a medical intervention.

Think about all of this and say out loud, "My body has let me down." Measure how true that feels on a scale of 0 to 10 where 0 is not true at all and 10 is completely true. Also notice any specific thoughts about your body that come up when you say it.

As you go through the tapping, feel free to personalize the script by adding or changing specific words or phrases that apply to you.

Tapping Script #2-1

There's my body – There it is – It's always been my body – And there have always been things wrong with it – I learned at a young age – As I became aware of my body – To reject parts of my body – That it was not good enough – Weak – Or deficient in some way – There had to be a time – When it didn't even occur to me – That there was something wrong with my body – My body was just part of me.

But I quickly learned – And it was a shock – That bodies can let you down – That there was something wrong with my body – And that's been proven to me – Because my body has let me down – It's really let me down – The way it looks – The way it acts – It's caused me pain – Suffering – Embarrassment – Humiliation.

I've been insulted – Laughed at and talked about – And I criticize my body too – There's something just not good enough – Ugly, broken – Not perfect – Not even close – And I can see it so clearly – I am looking right at those imperfections – And they are glaring – Ugh! – The truth is – It's not the body I really want – Why would I want to be – Super aware of my physical body? – I don't want to be in this body – I don't really like it – And that is just the truth – It's let me down – It's caused me suffering – I've been at war with this body – At times I have hated my body.

I've tried to negotiate with this body – I have even punished my body – I've tried to fix it – With willpower – Or meanness – Others have tried to fix it – And I just can't get there – So many things wrong with my body – And some of them truly feel unforgivable – Unforgivable – The truth is I reject my body – I reject my physical body – I want to love it – Sure, I want to love myself – But it's hard to love my physical body – Why would I want to be more *conscious of it? – I totally reject my physical body – And I am right about this – And I don't want to be talked out of it.*

Take a deep breath and notice how true the words felt for you.

If the words still ring true, tap through the script again. If you feel sad, just be with that. It means you are beginning to feel compassion for yourself.

Truthfully, we just spoke a lot of negativity. If you read the words without doing the visualization and tapping, you might think that saying these harsh words is harmful. Yet for some of us, these are the words that go through our heads all the time. It's eye-opening when we say our thoughts out loud and hear how negative they can be.

If you feel worse after tapping through that script, keep tapping and stay with it. It means you've hit on something that you've tried extremely hard not to feel. Starting to feel it can be emotional and come with a rising fear of being overwhelmed, but keep tapping! These are emotions and pain rising through your system that you can finally voice, hear, honor, and release. Holding them down helped you cope at times in your life, but it also keeps the pain locked down inside of you. It's time to let that go and move into healing.

If you notice you are tapping through the script and you believe the words feel true but you don't feel anything at all or you "go blank," you have disassociated from the experience. It's as if your mind said, *Nope, not going there!* and protectively shut down your rising feelings. Notice whether this is something you do often, as this might be how you dissociate, or leave your first chakra and go up into the safety of your thinking mind.

If that happens, tap and recite the following mini-script.

Mini Tapping Script #1: To bring you back into your body

I refuse to feel this – I refuse to be in my body – It's not safe – I refuse to deal with these issues – I don't want to have a body – I would rather not have a body – I don't want to be in my body at all.

That should bring you back into your body, and you will know pretty quickly why you don't want to be in it. Typically, the feelings start to rise and are uncomfortable, so keep tapping and breathing. One of the hardest emotions to tolerate and honor can be deep sadness.

Dissociation: The Big Disconnect

Dissociation is a term used to describe how people mentally disconnect from themselves and even their identity. It's akin to the freeze response, where our mind leaves our present experience. People will dissociate during serious trauma—even feel as if they are out of their body. They can do the same after a traumatic event. Many people with PTSD suffer from dissociation. It's the mind's way of not having to relive a terrifying experience.

When we dissociate from our first chakra (the body), the culprit can be a highly traumatic event or a series of smaller traumas we've felt over the course of a lifetime. By the time we're adults, we've learned how to effectively turn off some of our feelings.

Keep tapping through the above script and mini-script until the feelings are no longer overwhelming. Know that as you tap on the acupuncture points, you are rewiring your nervous system and releasing painful emotions so you no longer have to carry them around.

Check in again with the sentences "My body has let me down" or "My body is unforgivable," and see where you are now. Has the intensity has come down a bit?

We're going to do more tapping on this, so take a deep breath.

Tapping Script #2-2

Maybe I feel a little better – Maybe I feel worse – This is awful – Tuning into my body is terrifying – I actually do not want to go there – It's reminding me that I don't feel safe – At a core level – That I'm not in control at a core level – That I am vulnerable and weak – At a very basic level – I don't want to feel that – This is terrible – It reminds me that I'm weak – That I'm vulnerable – To the opinions and judgments of others – That I'm physically not capable of certain things – Not as strong as I want to be – Not as powerful as I want to be – Not as capable as I want to be – Tuning into my body reminds me – That I'm insecure – Totally insecure – And that I have a ball of shame that lives in me – All the time.

I am wired for fear, unsafety, and danger – And it's running in me all the time – I do not want to be in my body – I do not want to feel all this emotion – All this emotion, grief, pain – A lifetime of sadness – All focused on my body – If I let myself feel this – It could be a volcano – A river of tears – A river of sadness – Or maybe an unending well of fear – I really don't want to feel all this.

It's okay – It's just energy and it's moving – It's releasing and flowing – I've tightened up against it my whole life – My physical muscles have tried to contain it – My mind has been managing this – Holding down the lid – I'm moving that energy – That sadness, grief, disappointment, fear – It feels good to move that energy.

I totally honor myself right now – In this hard work that I'm doing – Because I'm never going to be the same – I'm never going to be the same after this moment – I'm moving this energy – It doesn't feel great, but every cell of my body is rejoicing right now – As I cry a river of tears – Every cell in my body is rejoicing with lightness – Every cell in my body is being washed by that river – The truth is I'm alive – This is my body – I like being alive – I'm glad I have a body – I'm honoring that today at a very basic level – I honor my body.

All this energy moving – I'm so open to lightening this up – Letting this go – Releasing, unblocking, and unwinding this flow of energy that's been stuck – Letting it flow up and out from my entire energy field – My nervous system and every cell of my body releasing.

Take a deep breath and notice how you're feeling right now. Notice how present you are. If you're still feeling your emotions flowing, know that it's okay. This is how your emotions and energy are supposed to move—up and out as they are voiced and heard with compassion.

If you let this energy move, if you voice it and let it clear, on the other side of that is a whole new way of being. It is a shift into being more loving, compassionate, and caring toward your body and more attentive and honoring of your pain, emotions, and needs.

Use this last round of tapping to continue to come into and experience your body in a refreshingly positive way.

Tapping Script #2-3

All this intensity, wow – My eyes are really open right now – To what I've been carrying in my body – What I've been blaming my body for – What I've been hating about myself – And it's not actually all of me – It's a piece of me – There's a part of me that runs this program – That runs this wounding – That runs this criticism of my body.

It's like a record player – It's like a recording – It was created in the past – Other people put their voice on the recording – Situations added to it – I've never even really questioned this recording – This part of me that's like a recording – It's been running and I've assumed it was real – That it was me – That it was the truth.

My eyes are open now – And I'm now observing – That there's a part of me – That actually decided at very young age to reject myself – And not feel these hard, vulnerable feelings – Probably to protect myself – I must have figured out – That if I hate and reject myself first – I'm less vulnerable – Or maybe that was what I learned I deserved.

I'm observing this now – And seeing how often it runs – It's running a lot – It's been running as if it's the truth – And I'm now seeing that it might not be the truth – That I might have a space here to make a choice – As I observe it, it weakens – As I observe it, I become conscious – And in the gift of consciousness, I can make a choice – To be more loving to myself.

The truth is that here in this moment – I am not broken – I am completely safe – I am whole, and I am alive.

My entire first chakra – Alive, vibrant, powerful – I honor my body – My body and I have a lot of work to do here – And I'm open to doing it – The truth is, in the here and now, I am a miracle – I am alive – I want to be alive and this is my body – I don't understand it – But I'm open to feeling my body in a way I never have before – Listening to what it is telling me – I am open to feeling my feelings – With more kindness than ever before – Even feeling my sadness and weakness – With more love and understanding.

Take a deep breath. Notice again how you're feeling.

If you are still experiencing intense emotions, repeat the last round of tapping until you feel calmer. The goal in this last tapping round is to anchor this moment of consciousness, to observe that your habitual negative self-talk isn't the truth. Once you reach that state, sit in that for a bit, take a deep breath, and simply notice your breathing. Then notice your hands and your feet. They may be pulsing with energy. Picture the image of pain, sadness, and other hard emotions and memories rising up and out as you hear them, bless them, and honor them one by one.

After a few minutes, close your eyes and picture that mirror again and notice your reflection. Is anything different? What distortions—a magnified "imperfection" or other flawed perception—in that fun-house mirror have shifted? Can you see more of your actual beauty and radiance? What if that is the real you? What if you have been beautiful and worthy all this time? Yes, breathe into that, and let your glorious energy radiate!

NEXT STEPS . . .

This week tune into the messages from your body and your emotions, whether they are intuitive or about the need for care, rest, nourishment, or pleasure. Catch those moments when you feel anxious or uncomfortable and write them down. Journal about what you did to listen to and meet that need for your body, even if meeting that need isn't possible in that very moment. With practice you will create a new habit of listening to your body and allowing your emotions to be felt and moved in a way that strengthens your first chakra and heals the past.

Visit www.unblockedbook.com/chapter3 for an extra tapping experience and discussion to enhance this chapter.

CHAPTER 4

HEALING THE ANXIOUS ENERGY PATTERN

"Who, me? Anxious? Naaah, not me. Maybe a little stressed, though!"

For many people being stressed out or under a lot of pressure is a badge of honor at certain times, especially when on the job. Many of us are wired to start out the day filled with a hum of anxious energy, regardless of external pressures. Some people wake up grumbling, already irritated at things they are picturing will happen that day and how frustrating it will be. A blocked first chakra leaves us feeling unnecessary anxiety most of the time.

Each of us operates at a daily baseline of fight or flight. It is important to recognize our baseline stress level because even moderate levels of stress can have a *massive* impact on health, day-to-day life, and ability to be in focused action.

Stress takes energy away from the immune, fertility, and hormone systems (the adrenal glands in particular), and it taxes digestion. Beyond that, and what most people don't realize, is that being in any level of the stress response wastes *huge* amounts of time because we are missing out on our most brilliant creative capabilities and mental focus. Instead our attention is scattered, routinely jumping from the task at hand, and our thinking is myopic, rigid, and fear based. At very high stress levels, it is as if we were trying to think clearly with a brain injury. No wonder we struggle to get certain things done!

The stress-response aspect of the first chakra takes even spiritually advanced people by surprise because it boils down to how we *really* operate on a daily basis. Are we frenetic, scattered, dependent on caffeine, and always running out of time? Are we frozen and ineffective, worried about "not being there yet," and wondering how we're going to get everything done and do it well? Or are we in the flow and taking joyful, excited, and focused action?

In case you need more motivation, I explain it to my clients this way: Imagine that stress response exists on a scale of 0 to 10, with 0 being totally at peace and 10 being highly stressed. At every degree past 0, you become that much less efficient, less effective, and less brilliant at everything you do. The good news is that turning stress, fear, and anxiety down even a few points means we shift into our smartest, most powerful, and most effective selves. And as we come out of the stress response, the relaxation response takes over and returns all our bodily functions to increasingly normal levels, boosting the immune system.

To get started we're going to dive into the important work of understanding and determining your average "walking around" level of stress as well as what happens to that level when you start tuning into important tasks you need to take action on.

HEALING EXPERIENCE #3: HEALING THE ANXIOUS ENERGY PATTERN

Setup Visualization #3-1

Take a breath and tune into your body. Close your eyes and go down into your body. One way to do that is to put your hands on your abdomen right under your rib cage. Imagine that, as you breathe in, you're not breathing through your mouth but directly into your heart. Take a few breaths that way and then imagine breathing in even lower into the core of your body, right behind your hand.

Feel the soles of your feet where they're touching the floor, and the chair supporting you.

Now imagine you can see on the movie screen of your mind a picture of you, sitting somewhere you typically sit at home. Maybe it is even an image from earlier today or a recent time you sat down to work on something important or were thinking about things in your life. First, just notice how you look in that picture—from the expression on your face to your body language. How does that version of you look? Sometimes we are surprised to notice how tired or stressed or sad we look, so really tune in. On a scale of 0 to 10, with 0 being totally at ease and 10 being panic-level stress, what number best describes your stress level?

It's important to self-assess your stress level so you know your baseline, or what I call your "walking around number." Many people are above 5, and I often hear 8 and 9 from people who never really thought about it before. Ask yourself whether anyone around you has any idea that your inner charge is that high. Too often the answer is no. We walk around looking sure and collected but are anxious and stressed and alone with the feeling, doing our best to contain it, hide it, and live with it.

Next, bring into this picture something that represents a big goal you have or something big you are working on or need to work on—something that is very important to you. Maybe you see it as a giant sign over your head with your goal written on it, or as a huge floating to-do list, or stacks of stuff piled in front of you. See what happens to your stress level on that same scale of 0 to 10 when you hold this in mind.

Note how that external list or goal might trigger some self-talk that increases your stress response by whipping up more fear. These fast-rolling thoughts might sound something like, *Oh, my gosh. What is wrong with me? I need to get this done. I need to figure this out. I should have had this done already.* All of these thoughts are driven by fear, even the smart-sounding ones. They're driven by a first chakra that has moved into survival mode in a very unhelpful way.

Now try this imagination experiment: Look at yourself again and see your nervous system as your body's electrical system. See all the nerves as if they were wiring pulsing with electric energy that flows from your spinal column to every limb and organ of your body, all the way up to your brain. See how your nervous system looks when stressed and note what is happening in your body and in your mind. Imagine you could somehow see the chemical side as well—stress hormones dispersing through your body, preparing you to fight, flee, or freeze as your mind goes blank.

Take a few moments to journal what you see. Write down your stress-level number as well as any aha moments or emotions that are coming up from visualizing yourself this way.

Take a deep breath and get ready to tap through the points.

Tapping Script #3-1

There I am – Anxious, stressed – I see that look on my face – I know what that means – I am stressed – And maybe overwhelmed and a little sad – Maybe I am exasperated and irritated – I see it in my body in this picture – And I can see what my mind is doing – I am observing my mental energy – And it is not "in the flow" – It is scattered – Thinking of too many things at once – Worrying about other things at the same time – Then yelling at myself too – Wow, no wonder I am not totally focused – And I am holding myself tight – My muscles tense – Neck, jaw, shoulders tight – I am holding myself up – Holding it together – Or maybe I am just holding on – I see and feel it in my body, my muscles, my energy.

I honor my inner fight-flight-freeze-bond response – I honor my primitive survival brain – I honor this fear response in my system – This ancient, inborn response wired into my genetics – For survival from times when survival was physical – Kill or be killed; fight or be eaten – I honor that my nervous system – Is running this survival program automatically – Causing physical changes in my body – And anxious energy in my thinking – This does not support me – It has become chronic – Because I'm walking around at this number – Which means the danger never goes away – The danger never goes away from me – At some level, I'm always on alert – Always on guard – Never safe to relax – Never a safe time to let go – Or let down and let out this holding of stress – Even when I sleep, I have to be on guard – I'm just going to honor that.

Post-Tapping Visualization #3-1

Take a deep breath. Close your eyes and look at the picture of you again. It should look a bit calmer. If not, tap through that round again. Notice whether any of the words triggered some sadness. This is very common, as you suddenly have a wave of self-compassion and understanding. When you look calmer in the picture, usually you feel calmer and more centered and balanced. Instead of your first chakra driving fear energy up through all your other chakras to your head, you now have more access to the wisdom of your heart.

From this energy, look at the picture again and tune into the biggest stressors floating around you—whether a live situation or big step you need to take to reach an important goal. What is really going on underneath your stress? What worries or fears are swirling around in your head? Fill in the blanks: "I am afraid ______ will happen . . . and that will feel ________." Finding out what is really at stake for you, or naming the internal fear at play honestly, is crucial to the healing process.

Next, notice what harsh words you might habitually be saying to yourself about the situation and what you are doing, not doing, or should be doing. This is the added internal pressure we put on ourselves—criticism or perfectionism—that escalates the stress.

Let's begin tapping again.

Tapping Script #3-2

There I am – And I see more of what is really going on – I am worrying more than I realize – There are things that actually feel risky – As if there is a lot at stake for me – That I haven't been aware of – There is real fear that is driving some of my stress – Fear of failing – Fear of things getting worse – Fear that nothing will change – Fear of being criticized – Something feels risky – There is a lot at stake – And I am pretty unforgiving about that – I am actually pretty hard on myself – And that is taking a toll – Adding to my stress – Increasing my anxious energy.

I can see that some of my anxiousness comes from my childhood – My first chakra wiring since childhood – From painful, scary experiences – From the many times that I was alone with being afraid – And things that I learned as truth about my safety in this world – I totally get it – And some of it comes from my big goals – My intention to step up and out – And the pressure I put on myself about that – Both trigger this primitive fear response – Which does not support me, not in the slightest – I totally honor that – And with new eyes and compassion – I honor all the ways fear gets in my way.

Take a breath and feel into your body.

Post-Tapping Visualization #3-2

How did it feel to see and honor that fear? What new insight do you have about how your mind-body system works? Do you feel any self-compassion?

Tune into the picture of you again and see how you look now. First, do you have a bit more understanding about your anxiety or what might be keeping you stuck and unfocused? This alone will help reduce the pressure you feel from any negative self-talk. But also notice how you look now. Most people report that they look calmer, grounded, and more present. It's common to suddenly see yourself enthusiastically taking action or even have a great idea pop up while you are tapping!

You can use either of those two previous rounds of tapping and this process of visualizing yourself every day to shift your stress response in the moment. Strangely, it is easier and more accurate to find out how we are feeling by imagining ourselves and *seeing* it instead of feeling it directly.

This final, positive round of tapping is designed to bring in even deeper shifts.

Tapping Script #3-3

It is my intention to shift out of the stress response – Into more calm in my body – A more centered state – Into more clarity and focus – Presence of body and presence of mind – So I'm bringing in some new understanding – I'm bringing in some new consciousness – To the most primitive unconscious part of my system – To my first chakra consciousness – To my automatic nervous system – There is no bear chasing me – I am not in life-threatening danger – I'm in my body – In this present moment – I am whole – I am safe – I am here – I am safe – I'm okay – The scary things are simply thoughts – Thoughts and ideas – Worries – Not about being killed – But about emotional pain – And I'm just going to honor that – I am open to feeling and holding my fears with kindness – My fears of experiencing emotional pain – Disappointment, upset, loss, criticism – I'm open to feeling and holding my fears with love – There is actually a lot at stake, and I am feeling it – All of my fears – But I'm not needing to fight – I am not needing to run – I don't need tense muscles – I don't need to brace for danger – The army in me gathering for a fight – Can stand down – This is peacetime – I am safe in my home.

My primitive brain has had this confused – And I get it – I honor that this is new information – New, surprising information to my survival brain – And I'm bringing it up anyway – I am safe – I will be safe – I am in my body, safe in this space – Giving my nervous system permission to stand down – To rest, to restore – To shift to a new level of calm in my system – A new concept of calm in my system – A new permission to be calm in my system – A new awareness of calm in my system – A new experience of calm in my system – A new understanding – It's time; it's okay for calm in my system – Dropping down now – One or two points into calm, calm in my system.

And that filters through my entire being, my physical body – More relaxed – Calmer heart and deeper breathing – My mind spacious

– Calm and clearer – And from this place of safety – My mind can be open and creative – My emotions become resilient – My physical being calming down one or two points – And entering a state of flow – Being in the zone – More centered, focused, and present – Thinking more clearly, more expansively – More brilliantly.

Take a deep breath. Check in with your body. How does it feel? Is energy moving? What do you notice?

If you notice an increase in anxiety, that's just the primitive part of your brain arguing against this new affirmation of safety. If needed, tap through the above script again.

NEXT STEPS . . .

Your assignment for the next week or two is to tap through a short script every day. This is a little challenge that will buffer your daily average level of stress and anxiety and make a *huge* difference in your life. You can use this quick exercise to relax or to heighten mental performance, including focus and creativity. Take a few minutes and tap to the above script, or you can simply tap through the points and say the following as many times as you'd like:

Mini Tapping Script #2: To reduce stress

All this stress and anxiety in my body – All this stress and energy I am carrying and holding – All this racing in my head – All this anxiety in my system – I am just going to honor it.

That's it! You can add more words, but it doesn't have to be fancy. You can add positive affirmations if you choose, but that basic simple tapping—even tapping without words—will cause a major overall shift to your state of being. This is the start of rewiring your brain and nervous system to operate in a calmer, more grounded way. You are also learning how to notice your anxiousness and lovingly attend to it so it can be soothed. This rebuilds your first chakra into one that is more solid and resilient. By tapping every day, you will see a consistent impact.

Visit www.unblockedbook.com/chapter4 for an extra tapping experience and discussion to enhance this chapter.

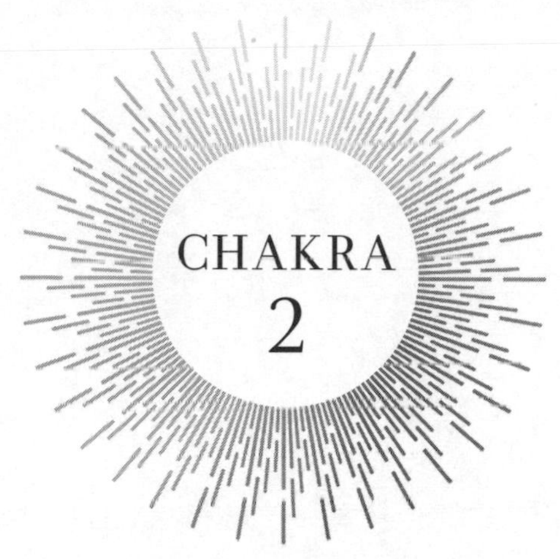

THE POWER OF POWER—HEALING THE SACRAL CHAKRA

Forget "follow your passion"
—*lead* with your passion!
All manner of miraculous inner gifts
and outer resources will *rise up*
and manifest to support you.

CHAPTER 5

RECLAIMING YOUR FUEL FOR MOTIVATION, ACTION, AND CHARISMA

Picture a huge dam hidden in a jungle. Made of boulders and rocks, the dam stops up a raging river. Downriver lies a village. Its residents have long forgotten who built the dam, and they never question why it's there. All they know is how difficult life has been due to a short supply of water. Some villagers work hard to grow crops and collect drinking water for everyone but to no end. Others sit on the sidelines; they've all but given up. Everyone is thirsty and starving. They have no energy. They are barely surviving.

If you were to bring the villagers to the dam, the only thing they would know for sure is that if the dam were to burst, it would unleash a destructive force. The entire village and all its people would be overwhelmed in one fell swoop. At best daily life would be paralyzed—changed forever. At worst the village would cease to exist.

That would be true if the dam suddenly burst open. But what if the dam were thoughtfully, carefully, and safely dismantled? What if the villagers started removing pebbles and small stones until the flow of water into the village was twice as strong? Immediately, the villagers would be energized, knowing they now had a chance to improve their lot. Everyone would feel better, stronger, and more vibrant and positive at the thought of moving from drought to abundance, hunger to health.

With this newfound strength, joy, and hopefulness, the villagers might ask themselves *what else* they could do with the power of this river. If they carefully open up more of the dam, they could contain and direct the river as a bigger energy source to charge up and energize the village. Suddenly, things that had seemed impossible would simply become a choice about how to direct this infinite source of abundance, physical well-being, and raw energy into advancement, growth, expansion.

In this metaphor the village represents you. The river is your second-chakra energy. The dam that is restricting your energy was mostly built in childhood, during now long-forgotten moments when you learned that expressing aspects of your second chakra was not safe. Every boulder, rock, and pebble in that dam is built with the rules you learned growing up that say it is not safe for you to have this big, potent energy.

Characteristics of the Sacral Chakra

Located just above the Root Chakra in the sacrum is the second chakra, or the fire that animates us. It's our drive—the fuel we need to lift us off our first-chakra foundation and move us to take action in the third chakra. Where the first chakra is characterized as solid, the second chakra is liquid, feeling, and sensory, and so I call it the river of life. It's where we get to *feel* our aliveness, own our power, understand our true needs and desires, and accept the more tender parts of ourselves.

The Sacral Chakra is vital to our well-being, yet it's grossly misunderstood. It usually only gets credit for sexual and creative energy. Important? Yes. All there is to the Sacral Chakra? No! The second chakra is the seat of *all* of our rising needs, wants, and desires that go beyond basic safety and survival, including the need to feel powerful, important, special, self-actualized, and celebrated for our gifts and talents.

The second chakra is rising empowerment energy that compels us to act on our desires. It's also the receiving chakra, where we ask for what we want or need and wait for it with arms wide open.

When second chakra energy is flowing, we *know* ourselves and what we want at any given moment because we *feel* ourselves—our deepest needs and desires. We are all at once authentically joyful, fun, powerful, confident, humble, charismatic, caring, sensitive, and vulnerable. We are *dynamic* and exude an irresistible presence and energy that others feel as real, passionate, and bubbling with aliveness.

BUILDING THE DAM: ANGER (POWER) AND NEEDINESS (VULNERABILITY) DENIED

What exactly is this dammed-up river of second-chakra energy? It's everything we gave away when we learned that it was not safe or acceptable to be angry or needy.

In Chapter 1 we talked a lot about how the nervous system gets wired at the first chakra so we feel either fearful or safe and assured that we will be supported as we change and grow. The same concept applies to our *feelings, desires, needs, and impulses to act on them* in the second chakra. These second-chakra impulses are core to who we are as individuals. They are how we express our uniqueness.

Anger and neediness are two big pieces of our emotional puzzle at the second chakra. When we first express these emotions as children, we're usually doing it for good reason—we have an impulse to meet a need, even if it's to throw a tantrum as a way to say, *Hey, this doesn't feel fair!* These two pieces of the second chakra build on our first-chakra foundation of believing we deserve and have the right to want things we want and to get angry if we are wronged. But anger and neediness carry some very negative connotations and aren't always well received by our tribe. We're told to stop whining and to "knock it off."

As unattractive as anger and neediness might sometimes appear to be, both of these energies are vital. Both are meant to fuel motivation, courage, action, and even charisma. Without them we are incomplete. So we need to learn about their true power, break down the dam, and take them back.

When expressed maturely, anger and neediness are essential pieces of our rising power. These rising, felt energies compel us to set a healthy boundary or simply ask for what we want or deserve—even if it's just a hug. They build in intensity at times to *empower* us to speak out when something is unfair, or to boldly ask to receive something even when the act leaves us feeling momentarily vulnerable.

When we're led to believe that anger is always scary and bad, we deny what would someday grow into a mature expression of power. When the message is that it's weak or selfish to ask for what we want or need, as adults we will refuse to ask for anything that makes us appear weak or selfish. *We're left, then, to ignore what we really want, suppress our rising desires and impulses (some of which are unique to us), and only do and want things that we feel are safe.*

It all starts with hot-stove moments.

HOT-STOVE MOMENTS

The village dam is an accumulation of "hot-stove moments," or the times when our rising desires and impulses were met with abrupt shame and punishment by our primary caregivers. When, as a young child, we naively ask for something or follow an impulse and are met with anger or punishment, it feels painful and shocking, much like touching a hot stove. We quickly learn that denying some of our innate needs and desires—literally holding back—is safer than expressing them. We don't want to get burned again.

Month by month and year by year, as our second chakra begins to develop and compels us to explore and experience our world, we become increasingly independent and active. Some of our new actions are encouraged and applauded, but not every action of reaching out to test the waters is welcome.

Toddlers, for instance, have a seemingly tireless river of energy to move, touch, and experience things. They start saying *no!*, demanding and grabbing things, getting angry, and experiencing the energy charge it creates in their parents. They also start performing, laughing, helping, and hugging more . . . and taking in the reactions from their parents.

At second-chakra phases of growth and behavior, this energy brings kids headlong into new sets of tribal rules and consequences for breaking those rules. These rules and consequences can direct this flowing second-chakra energy in affirming ways with consequences that act as boundaries to contain the powerful force of the second chakra. This might sound like, "It's not okay to hit and grab," followed by a time-out, or the rules and consequences can lead to hot-stove moments that have lifelong, crippling implications.

Cost of a Weak Second Chakra

- Finding difficulty truly owning your power
- Feeling guilty or anxious about being "too powerful" or "too attractive"
- Trying to never to be angry and priding yourself as being "better than that"
- Being angry and in battle all the time with others and/or the self in the form of self-sabotage
- Overthinking and idolizing thinking as more important than feelings
- Finding difficulty feeling joy and connection

- Experiencing patterns of total fear and avoidance of vulnerability due to expecting betrayal and abandonment
- Shutting down of sexual energy and/or periods of excessive sexual energy

Benefits of a Strong Second Chakra

- Channeling raw life-force energy that will be felt by you and others as personal power, passion, charisma, creative ability, and sexuality
- Experiencing the massive charge of raw life-force energy spurring and emboldening you to act and go for what you really want and deserve
- Feeling *you—who* you are, what you're drawn toward, and what you truly want
- Feeling your heart opening and allowing more love, intimacy, and vulnerability into your relationships, while setting healthy boundaries
- Allowing your passion, energy, and ups and downs to be felt by others
- Being willing to be vulnerable, flawed, and human
- Being able to feel your emotions, needs, pleasure, and joy, and having a willingness to celebrate you

THE SHAME GAME

No parents are perfect, but if parents use shame or anger consistently as a consequence, it sends the message that you are "bad"—instead of just correcting specific actions that are problematic. Shaming always has the *How dare you!* element, which conveys to a child that there is something wrong about the fact that they even tried to do whatever they did.

The trying is inextricably tied to the natural second-chakra impulse of *I want and should be able to have that,* which compels us into action. So it is also a hot-stove lesson in how shockingly wrong a child's assumption is about what they have the right to want and their power to act on it. The result is that the mistake or misstep is never "undone." Even if the mess is cleared and apologies are given, the sting and shock of shame remains burning in the pit of the stomach.

This is where a child first hears their needs, wants, desires, hurts, fears, or anger described with words that convey how bad and therefore unwanted and unacceptable these core impulses (i.e., who they are) seem to their parents. They learn that their fear makes them a weak baby, their need makes them selfish, their desire for attention makes them spoiled, their innocent mistakes make them stupid, their anger makes them an arrogant brat, their desire for freedom makes them lazy, and their desire for pleasure makes them disgusting.

When parents react with *How dare you!* shame, children feel in their bodies the danger in the charged reaction of anger and frustration or disappointment and withdrawal. It feels like a shock, an attack; or an unexpected, unforeseen new danger as important as life or death. A young mind must scramble to figure out this new type of rule so they can avoid this painful new type of punishment.

Shame usually triggers the bond response as a survival adaptation. To better understand why, think of being held hostage by a bank robber. To stay alive we might appease the attacker or even offer to help them escape and promise not to tell the authorities. Now imagine an explosively angry parent and a child who acts in a loving, protective, caring, and complimentary manner to stay out of harm's way.

But in a more subtle way, being shamed will cause a child to contain their rising second-chakra natural impulses so they don't break this new rule and upset their parents. With repeated reinforcement we will find ourselves hardwired at the nervous-system level to forever feel a rush of anxiety and shame with any impulse that has been labeled as shamefully bad or unacceptable in our family.

Let's explore four different scenarios of how second-chakra impulses are handled in different families and the impact of each. These are composites that merge the stories of many of my clients. Which most relates to your history?

Scenario One: Mary's Story

Mary was extremely close to her father. She barely remembers getting in trouble as young girl, but she does remember some serious heart-to-hearts with Dad. He was tuned into and good with her feelings, whether she was angry or sad or anxious. She remembers thinking he had some magic power to know what was going on with her. As a new mom, Mary asked her dad how he handled her when she was "naughty."

He told her that, first, he tried to "nip things in the bud" or "head things off at the pass." This was his way of saying he came in early to check in and redirect. When this failed he used time-outs or simple consequences such as an apology that "made things all better." He said that though he wasn't ever perfect, his goal was first and foremost that she grow in confidence even when she got into trouble.

He got his wish, as Mary is always ready to take on new challenges and is resilient when things don't go as planned. She believes in herself, has courage when she needs it, and has become an excellent leader in her career. Whenever she feels off or struggling, she knows she can just ask for help from her father, friends, or partner.

Scenario Two: Joan's Story

Joan doesn't remember a lot of her childhood infractions, but she vividly remembers her dad exploding in anger and frustration. Sometimes she and her siblings saw it coming, and other times it came out of nowhere. He would yell, throw things at the nearest kid, and storm around the room. Even as an adult, she finds it upsetting and emotional to talk about these scenes and how scared she felt. Joan learned to tiptoe through the house, trying to be as quiet and as small as possible to avoid triggering her father.

As an adult Joan struggles to progress in her career because just the thought of stepping up and being more seen fills her with anxiety and self-doubt. It doesn't feel safe, so she has spent years, as she says, "hiding." She also spent many years feeling trapped in a relationship with an angry, demanding man whom she found herself tiptoeing around.

Scenario Three: Tom's Story

Tom was raised by his grandparents, whose favorite expression was "Know your place." One day he came home from school clearly glowing with a big smile on his face. "What's gotten into you?" they asked. He couldn't wait to proudly tell them how he had won the class spelling bee and that the teacher gave him a gold star. He remembers the shock of what happened next. "Well, now, I guess you think you're better than us, don't you? You think you are so smart? Nobody likes a know-it-all."

He was not physically hit, but it sure felt like a slap in the face. He believes he just froze in that moment. He can still recall that awful sick feeling of shame and humiliation in the pit of his stomach. Tom experienced many hot-stove moments like this over his childhood. Each *Who do you think you are?* moment reminded him that believing in himself, feeling good about himself, or acting as if he deserved something would result in the painful punishment of shaming.

Tom learned to squelch his good feelings about himself quickly by telling himself things like *I am such a loser.* That worked well to make sure he never acted that "full of himself" again. Throughout his young adult life, he struggled with feeling deeply flawed, broken, and not good enough—even while he excelled in school.

As he began his career as an EMT, he was often treated unfairly and underpaid, but he never really got mad. He just kept his head down and took it. He worked incredibly hard without asking for much and therefore never got much.

At times he would have a surge of energy and ideas and would do something new, exciting, and bold. But his successes were short-lived. He would start to feel like a fraud, wondering, *Who do I think I am?* He would start to worry that people were going to be jealous or attack him or think he was arrogant. In the end he always self-sabotaged any reward he got or progress he made, once again proving to himself that he really was just not good enough.

Scenario Four: Kristin's Story

Kristin grew up in a good home with two loving, smart, successful, and busy parents who set high standards for their daughter. If Kristin failed to meet certain expectations, she got "the look." If she made a mistake or got a bad grade, her parents seemed shocked and let down that she didn't try harder or didn't care enough to get it right. Without saying a word, all her mother needed to do was give Kristin that steely, stern look, and the message was clear: *I am so disappointed in you.* She could feel the hurt.

Kristin barely ever cried as a child because she knew that was unacceptable. Any show of weakness, fear, or other emotional expression was ignored or met with an eye roll as her parents changed the subject or walked away. As an adult Kristin became a perfectionist but didn't take compliments well because, truth be told, she thought other people's standards were woefully low. She always knew she could have done better. She worked such long hours that she often became sick and burned out. Those times were the worst because she hated herself when she was unproductive and really hated having to let her husband take care of her. Though she achieved a lot, she never quite felt like she had "arrived" yet, so she could never let her foot off the gas pedal.

SOMETHING'S MISSING

What makes natural impulses, desires, needs, and emotions (and ultimately each of us) interesting is that they serve a purpose—they are energy with a message. The second chakra is a big level of consciousness, or awareness, and part of its job is to offer inner guidance. Being aware of what we need and feel is key to knowing ourselves and what will fulfill us. The costs of trying *not* to feel our feelings, needs, and wants for a lifetime are many and always result in feeling frustrated and empty on the inside. In quiet moments we will realize that something is missing, even when we are outwardly successful.

Rising desires and needs and feelings of "reactionary anger" (my term for anger that occurs in reaction to being wronged), frustration, or grief—examples of this pure life energy—are supposed to inform and empower us. Every desire and impulse, as well as the strong feelings that come with them, has something important to tell us about ourselves. Rather than accept these messages as guidance and part of who we are, we try to disown and not feel them.

The problem with our natural second-chakra impulses is that they never go away, and we know they are there. We will still feel our desire for attention, power, pleasure, and fun. We will still feel our fears and needs as well as our reactionary anger and rage that leans into hatred. This leaves us no other option than to harbor a secretive inner truth we must always hide from the world: At our core, there is something unacceptable about us. If others found out how bad and broken we really were, they'd be shocked and horrified. They would reject us. This is the insidious quality of shame. And it's what gives it staying power.

THE STAYING POWER OF SHAME

What starts out as parental shaming turns into adult self-shaming. We judge an impulse as our parents did, and that stops us in our tracks from whatever we were about to do for fear of how it will look. We don't base our life around a family rule that said

Tuesday was our night to wash the dishes. But we will be hypervigilant about never being seen doing something so "selfish and lazy" as that one time we left the dishes until morning and those unforgettable words hit us like a slap in the face. As adults, if we have a day where we feel like being "selfish and lazy," we won't allow it.

Self-shame effectively keeps us cooperating, being helpful, not needing much, acting humble, apologizing, playing small, and being obsessed with a fear of making mistakes (trying to be perfect). Self-shame ensures we act in a way so that no one is angered by us, no one disapproves of us, and no one can be disappointed in us. We shame ourselves into staying small. That way, and only that way, can we safely belong and thrive in the tribe.

But there is a price to pay for chronic shame. When used chronically to contain our natural impulses, self-shame will always trigger a reactionary angry—or anger fueled by the nervous system's stress response. For some this attack is directed at other people, such as the teenager who rebels against restrictive parents. For others it is a secret self-attack that leads to depressive self-loathing and self-blame. Author Anodea Judith calls this being "shame bound." Our second-chakra energy of desires, wants, and reactionary anger cannot rise up to fuel our actions because shame is beating it down.

Shame always takes us down at the second chakra, especially when it comes to feeling angry. Few people, for instance, admit that they have ever felt rageful. They'd be ashamed if others saw them that way. *How would people react if I were honest about these terrible, terrible feelings? If people knew what I was really like, they'd never talk to me again.* We assess ourselves like this all the time. We look at ourselves and think, *OMG, I'm horrible.*

This is especially hard when there is additional fear about who we would "look like." Clients will tell me, "I vowed to never be like my father. If I get angry, I will look just like him." I have also had many clients who feel their anger and believe it is their father's or mother's anger living in them, so they are afraid to express it. This means they can't honor it, listen to it, or understand it as their own anger that is rising up in reaction to something unfair.

And then there are those moments when we are painfully and unexpectedly blindsided with the reaction we fear most. I am referring to those moments when we feel courageous, allow ourselves to feel confident, and someone says, "Aren't *you* full of yourself?" Ouch. We're flooded with shame. We will immediately self-sabotage whatever it is we got all "high and mighty" about. That'll teach us to be so sure of ourselves or proud of our accomplishments or, God forbid, to ask for attention.

Everyone has their kryptonite. Being selfish used to be mine. All someone had to say to me was, "You're being selfish," and whatever boundary I was trying to set was washed away instantly. My words failed me, and my energy drained. I'd be so ashamed, I'd spend all my time proving I wasn't selfish—which usually meant acting like a doormat while people-pleasing.

I find that people have long forgotten why they started to judge pieces of themselves as bad, shameful, and unacceptable, but they are extremely invested in their secret self-shaming. To them it seems completely justified, based in real facts and evidence from their past, and the smart and correct thing to do. This is why it is important to see shame for what it really is—survival fear designed to stop you before you break family rules that are contrary to your natural, built-in human needs, desires, and wants.

How do you talk someone out of their deeply held and hidden places of shame? You don't. You have to use the tapping process. When we tap to voice, honor, and move our shame and other negative emotions, what's left behind is what we really want. It's the answer to all the questions we couldn't answer before. If this is making me so angry, what next? What do I need?

FIRE HOSE ON THE LOOSE: IMMATURE EXPRESSIONS OF THE SECOND CHAKRA

Second-chakra emotions, needs, and impulses are incredibly strong. If they are not allowed to be conscious, they will find unconscious ways to come through. Sometimes this manifests as uncharacteristically acting out in ways that shock others (and us!)

or in "losing it" with anger or breaking down. When this kind of rupture happens, it is never empowering and always replays our worst-learned fears about being embarrassed, humiliated, and ashamed of ourselves.

Every second-chakra impulse has a mature and an immature expression. Buried impulses are expressed immaturely. It's as if our empowerment energy were water coming through an active fire hose on the loose, swirling out of control with no firefighter to hold it in place, direct the powerful force of water, and put out the fire.

The second chakra unleashed as immature reaction can be destructive, like a bursting dam destroying a village. It can rage like a river through our system and drive compulsive behaviors and addictions that are impossible to control with logic or discipline regardless of how smart or goal oriented we are. Drug addiction, compulsive shopping or gambling, and physical abuse are all second-chakra issues of excess need with no healthy expression or direction.

Using willpower and extreme self-discipline to contain our powerful second chakra will not work. Eventually we will hit a point where we suddenly go overboard. This is always so traumatic to people that they go right back to trying to shame their needs and desires without ever learning how they move into maturity. This is exactly what I will be leading you to and through—the mature recognition, value, and expression of pent-up second-chakra energy so you can safely use your river of power without fear of blowing up your life.

One way to know whether our second chakra is blocked is to be aware of when we're acting from a place of emotional immaturity—or criticizing someone else who is. Ever look at someone and think, *Unbelievable—I would never ever act like that*? Maybe it's a friend who seems to be clamoring for attention by posting every single thing she does on social media. Maybe it's that guy at work who's always complaining and demanding more. Inside, we're sure that if we behaved like that, we'd look ridiculously needy, which for us would be committing a crime practically punishable by death.

I would never allow myself to be that way! is something we feel really sure and right about. It is annoying and sometimes embarrassing to witness someone acting out from a whiny, needy, immature place. That's easy to agree on. Yet the intensity of our critical reactions toward another's immature acting-out is a great clue to what needs we've been denying in ourselves—what we've learned is impossible to ask for but what we actually need. If we're criticizing another for needing too much attention, it's a sure bet we need some attention ourselves.

OH, GROW UP! MOVING INTO MATURE EXPRESSION OF THE SECOND CHAKRA

Ever noticed that *courage* contains the word *rage*, the feeling most of us try to hide from? *Rage*, when properly channeled, becomes out*rage*. Then it becomes cou*rage*. Anger and rage are important empowerment emotions that have mature and immature expressions. When expressed maturely, anger gives us the fuel we need to right a wrong or set a boundary and the courage to take action—all without completely losing control.

The mature expression of neediness is vulnerably voicing (or admitting to) our true needs, how important they are, and asking for them to be met no matter how embarrassing we worry they may sound and no matter how exposed admitting to them makes us feel. The trick to "growing up" is to own our anger and needs in every moment. And it is tricky, if only because many people would rather die than get mad or show "weakness." But when expressed maturely, anger and vulnerability are two of the most powerful emotions on the planet.

Most of my clients will argue until they're blue in the face that they aren't angry, and in all honesty, I used to say the exact same thing. Many people make a conscious effort to never show anger. They are actively afraid and judgmental of people who are angry, usually because they had an outwardly angry parent. They may never get overtly mad, but it usually surfaces as anxiety or depression. They aren't aware that they may have repressed angry feelings and, along with them, a piece of what makes them feel alive.

When we do get angry, it's for one reason and one reason alone: something felt unfair, either to us or someone we love or empathize with. When I read this simple truth years ago in *The Secret Language of Feelings* by author Cal Banyan, I could not refute it. Anger is always saying, *Hey, I don't like this. This feels unfair.* When something feels unfair, there's sure to be an unmet need buried underneath. That energy rises and fills us with the focus and increased energy to speak up, change something, or set a boundary.

Sometimes it takes an injustice outside ourselves to move our rage so we're willing to speak out (outrage) and take action to make a difference (courage). Mothers Against Drunk Driving is a perfect example. These parents were so outraged that their children died because intoxicated people were allowed to get behind the wheel of a car and, in effect, commit murder. This group had the courage to unite and change drunk driving laws nationwide. And they altered how entire generations look at drinking and driving.

Anger is supposed to come up to reveal the hurt and give us the charge to make a change. Tears, grief, and hurt are supposed to surface so we can be lovingly held by others and ourselves and express what we've lost but still need. When this fuel rises up to the third chakra, we muster up the courage to take action.

In a perfect world with no obstacles ever in our path, we don't need anger or courage or vulnerable expressions of need. Passion and desire drive us forward, and we simply ask for what we need and receive it. An even bigger bonus is if we have a strong first chakra. We don't question whether we have the right to desire something. We just let our passion drive us forward. In the real and imperfect world, where we don't always get what we need and life can be unfair, we rely on moments of anger and vulnerability to overcome barriers and adversity to get what we truly want.

The second chakra, then, is a place of opposites. Every need expressed immaturely buries a true, positive need. Every emotion expressed immaturely is telling us something hurts and is not fair. All these messages get to who we are at our core.

Once we start the tapping exercises, feelings and their messages become easier to recognize so we're far better at containing them not behind a hidden dam but with a healthy dose of consciousness.

HEALTHY CONTAINMENT

Just as the villagers feared the overwhelming torrent of the dam breaking, our stuck second-chakra emotions need to be handled carefully with healthy containment. This is where tapping becomes a useful and powerful tool. It releases emotion while returning us to a place of calm. Even when used in clients with severe PTSD, tapping does not retraumatize. In the process of healing and opening up our second-chakra empowerment energy, we will use tapping every step of the way to move forward in a safe, grounded way.

As we heal, the intensity of locked-away needs, hurts, and shame will start to subside and allow our second-chakra needs to move into adulthood. Instead of acting impulsively, having a tantrum, or completely shaming and shutting ourselves down, we are more present to calling in the need. Then we're able to run it through our head and heart and ask, *What do I really want?*

The goal is to express ourselves consciously—to draw from the consciousness of our upper chakras to know the difference between right and wrong, always seek a win-win situation, set boundaries that are fair, and learn the art of assertiveness and acceptance.

WALKING-GHOST SYNDROME

After listening to many clients over the years try to convince me they don't "need all that messy stuff" and that they just want to be smart and strong, it is my firm opinion that it is not okay to shut down, let go of, or ignore any piece of your second chakra. There's no piece of your second chakra that you could live without. It's every bit as crucial to your well-being as your body's vital organs. There is no piece of the multifaceted aspects of the second chakra that you can live without and be full-on alive, passionate, charismatic, and in your mission. When you look around, you see people who've chopped up and denied aspects of their second chakra. We don't have time for that. Life is only truly lived when we feel fully alive in every waking moment.

If you are denying your vulnerability, needs, ability to receive power, sensual experience of the world and other people, sexual energy, rage and anger energy—if you are denying any piece of that and saying, *I'm not going to experience that. Not okay, not acceptable,* you are half alive. The diagnosis for that is what I call Walking-Ghost Syndrome. People who aren't living through their second chakra are walking through life without feeling and without feeling alive. They chase stuff, achievements, or sexual partners to feel alive. They chase in the outside world what they want to feel on the inside. They chase buying things. They chase more achieving, and when they get there, they think, *I was supposed to feel something.* But they don't. Something is still missing.

So I invite you to recognize and trust. As you go through the upcoming Healing Experiences and feel the energy of this second chakra, you will feel all those impulses. Some of them you will choose not to act on, but the important thing is to feel them fully and express them maturely.

A RIVER RUNS THROUGH IT

Despite everything the Sacral Chakra promises to deliver, it can be a scary place for so many of us. The thought of opening the floodgates and suddenly reliving the pain associated with unfulfilled desires, needs, and impulses is terrifying. Added to that are the dammed-up "negative" feelings—all the years of anger, sadness, neediness, grief, regret, guilt, and shame that have been so snugly contained by the wall we've put up. We will do anything not to feel these painful emotions. Even if starving for courage, passion, and energy, all we can think of is how angry and vulnerable all those feelings would make us.

If someone suggested that we tear down the dam, or if those feelings started creeping up, we would feel anxiety followed by discouraging thoughts: *Why would I want to feel that? There's no point. Nothing is going to change if I feel it. Why would I want to cry? It might overwhelm me. I might go someplace that I'll never come back from. I won't be able to get anything done. I'll just feel anxious.*

No one wants to willingly go to that scary place, yet some of the emotions we want to feel the least are the ones that can empower us the most. Anger and any form of weakness or neediness are some of the big ones. By not acknowledging and moving the painful emotions, we don't get to experience the joyful, passionate, or exuberant ones either. They're all mixed up in that river together. The second chakra is about feeling everything from desire to rage, regardless of whether we judge these impulses to be good or bad. At the second chakra, feelings are fuel. All of them.

Tearing down the dam, even one pebble at a time, opens up a massive level of awareness and growth that can start a chain reaction. Life energy starts coursing through and busts open pieces of the dam until it creates a channel that slowly and manageably grows in size and force. Once this energy starts moving, we're suddenly excited. We feel a delicious, yummy, childlike joy. We feel like a kid again, ready with enthusiasm to go after what we want in this world. The pain we associated with our natural impulses fades away and eventually ceases to exist.

In the upcoming Healing Experiences, I'm going to lead you down a pathway of taking out pebbles and stones in a controlled, careful manner so we slowly open up the dam. We're going to move massive amounts of denied emotions in a safe and contained way, freeing up pure life-force second chakra energy.

Best of all it won't be scary. The village won't flood. We won't lose a single person. We will just liberate them one pebble at a time. When you're done opening up the floodgates—when you've voiced, honored, and moved all the old stuff that formed the dam in the first place—you'll *feel yourself* for the first time in a very long time.

Second-chakra work is like waking a powerful sleeping giant. It can get messy when shame, neediness, and anger pop up in response to what's going on in our life now. At first we might yell at everyone in the house, cry at the slightest offense, be overcome with anxiety, or cover ourselves in a blanket of shame. But that sleeping giant is nothing to fear. Waking it is exciting. Once we name the feeling and the need or desire, we feel it and own it and turn it into the beautiful energy of power and drive. With tapping it's totally manageable.

In the processes I'm going to lead you through in the next three chapters, we aren't going to just tap away anger and sadness and neediness. We're going to acknowledge their messages—their guidance—so we can reclaim our second chakra energy to meet our needs. Now let's start taking down the dam.

COMMENTARY BY DAVID RANIERE, PH.D.

I recall vividly a memory of my daughter from around the time she was two years old. It was a quiet, sunny early-Saturday morning during the summer. The world was still asleep, but we were up. I was following her with my cup of coffee as she made her way out of the house through the screen door. She stepped out onto the front porch, and with outstretched arms she faced the street as she loudly and excitedly announced, "I'm here!"

My sleep deprivation immediately gave way to lightness and ease, ushered in by the big sound of her young voice and the excited pitch and simple delight in her confident delivery. I looked over her head to see which one of our neighbors she was talking to, and I was amazed to discover that nobody was there. She was simply celebrating her arrival into that day, sending out a call for all to hear. This was to be her day, and it was going to be a great one because she was in it.

I forgot all about that cup of coffee in my hand as tears rolled down my face. What was making me cry? It had to do with how free and open she was, how unrestrained she was in her joyful expressiveness, and how completely absent shame was for her in that moment.

As a child I had always been careful not to make too much noise, and learned early on to be quiet, still, and go unseen. And here she was, being so "out there" and un-self-conscious in her excitement. She was feeling and extending herself openly toward the world from that place within herself, sending a strong, positive signal that set all sorts of good things in motion. What a way to start the day!

What my daughter did that morning is sadly the kind of thing we learn over time to stop doing. For all sorts of reasons and in all sorts of ways—some necessary and inevitable as part of the socialization process and others quite unfortunate and costly—we learn to restrict our range of emotional experience and how we express it. Freud's book on the subject, *Civilization and Its Discontents,* captures this concept well.

The truth of the second chakra is that we know ourselves through what we feel, and our wishes, needs, and desires are core to who we are. As Margaret describes, this includes vital elements of emotional life that tend to get a bad rap: the rising power of anger and the softness and vulnerability associated with our needs. Maintaining a sense of safety and belonging comes first, and we inhibit feelings, thoughts, and actions that pose a threat to our connections with others.

Inhibition is the dam that blocks the flow of our vital life energy. And inhibition takes many forms, including cautiousness, being quiet or still, taking up only a little space, trying to be invisible, not making any sudden moves, and being exceedingly gentle. But these efforts to keep us safe also carry and reinforce shame. The more passive forms of inhibition identified above are silent killers that may be rationally justifiable and so well integrated into one's operating system that they may not even appear to involve shame at all, but they do.

In contrast the more active form of self-shaming involves the vicious voice of the brutal inner critic who assaults the self with disparaging judgments and self-loathing. This form of shame can be easier to identify so long as you can separate yourself enough from its bullying tactics to recognize its brutality; if not, you will instead maintain that its judgments are accurate assessments and its beatings punishment you deserve.

In Chapter 1 I described the still-face effect and emphasized our rootedness in connection and how disruptions to it have a profound impact on the nervous system at the first chakra level. There the still-face effect is understood as a precursor to a shame response, experienced in the infant's body long before language and memory systems have fully developed. Here, at the second chakra level, a bit further down the developmental line, the young child has begun to use words and establish crude forms of logic that govern their understanding. Beliefs about the self are now "online" in cognitive form, surfacing long after they had been lived in bodily experience.

Shame-based beliefs during childhood and beyond sadly toggle between two renderings of the self: *I am too much*, and *I am not enough*. Patterned exchanges with others that carry those messages are now able to be encoded and translated in the cognitive realm using these kinds of words. These words calcify into beliefs, and these beliefs become the boulders that block the river of our emotional vitality.

In the tapping processes ahead, Margaret will gently approach that dam wall, and we will begin to carefully see how it's built and how to allow more of a current to pass through by taking away one stone at a time. The promise of second-chakra work is to step out on your own porch with outstretched arms and take delight as you extend yourself more fully into the world.

CHAPTER 6

THE POWER OF VULNERABILITY

"I would rather die than be needy or weak—but oh, yes, vulnerability is important!"

I hear this contradiction a lot. Although it has become more in vogue to talk about vulnerability as a strength, most people only see it working for other people. On the surface we love the idea of other people being able to feel our passion and how much we truly care. However, the actual work of trying to become more vulnerable by delving into our most soft and guarded places sends most people running for the hills. The whole concept sounds crazy if they've spent a lifetime trying to prove they are not weak, needy, sensitive, or emotional. For many people those are the very qualities they can't stand in others and wholly reject in themselves. This is what makes second-chakra work counterintuitive in concept and in practice. Yet counterintuitive we must be.

What is the promise in this strange type of work? Despite an almost-universal distaste for weakness, most of my clients will admit that they are not quite sure who they really are. They work hard and give and do a lot, yet there is an emptiness inside, a hollowness. Something is missing in their lives that they can't find or figure out, and they feel alone with that, even when in a relationship. And despite their epic giving and hard work, they never feel that they are getting the money, respect, attention, and love that deep down they have been hoping and waiting for.

This unsolvable problem is how I get clients to *try* second-chakra work. Instead of telling them I am going to help them be more vulnerable, I tell them this work will bring them all the things they are truly after in life. I can make that alluring offer because it is exactly what the second chakra is all about: the wants-and-desires side of the second chakra is the basis of their unique fire hose of empowerment energy. But instead of directly challenging the *I can never be weak* identity, we ease into the work by looking at the inner-child aspect of the second chakra.

This is where you need to go to start healing and discovering this most sacred and powerful but misunderstood aspect of your true self. It is like visiting with a side of you that not only knows what you really want but also has the rising energy of impetus you need to ask for and receive your wants and desires.

You've likely learned not to feel your true, deep needs and instead think a lot of thoughts about what is either more appropriate to want or what you can actually get. This is a trickle instead of a fire hose of the rising empowerment energy of passion, enthusiasm, and drive. The first step in second chakra work is to connect with your true needs and heal early pain that taught you not to feel them. We must visit a time when you learned as a young child that it was safer to avoid the pain and disappointment of feeling a desire that you've learned will never be fulfilled.

I PROMISE NOT TO MAKE YOU NEEDY!

Before we dive in, it is important to acknowledge that the second chakra is a place of extremes, and that's not what we're going for. No one wants to be *that* person—the one who is so consistently needy that they drain and exhaust everyone. This is the immature second-chakra expression of vulnerability and our fear of it can stop us from owning and expressing our true needs.

Working through the second chakra with tapping allows us to heal and bring balance to our second-chakra energy extremes. The needs we are afraid of can be voiced, heard, honored, and soothed as we tap with this intention. That is how we transform what you might call immature or over-the-top needs, desires, and reactions into more mature expressions of what we want in our life right now as adults. First and foremost, being vulnerable requires stepping out of our comfort zone—going outside the parameters set in our childhood about what is okay to admit to needing and feeling.

For example, a big fear around "neediness" is being afraid of overtly seeking attention. But the truth is, we are supposed to want and *need* certain attention. As adults we *need* to experience the good, celebratory feelings and joy of recognition and praise for our accomplishments. Deep down, of course we want praise! We want people to see our work, passion, care, and brilliance in a *Wow, you are amazing* moment. It feels good to be celebrated, and it is supposed to feel good. When we get this reward in the mix with other things around our accomplishments, our fulfillment drives our motivation more than willpower alone. We are charged up by the good-feeling loop and full of energy and passion to do more.

I have met many smart, hardworking people who are so defensive against feeling the need to be celebrated or be the center of attention that they go to great lengths to prove that they don't need it, want it, or think they are special. When praise and acknowledgment show up, they deflect and jump out of the spotlight. But in opening the second-chakra energy, everything changes. When those same people finally let down the wall and allow in a meaningful compliment, suddenly they admit that this is what they have always wanted and hoped for but never let themselves have.

So I invite you to wonder what it has cost. What has this lifetime of actions designed to *prove* you deserve something, while quietly *hoping* to receive it, cost you? What would it be like to ask for exactly what you want, with your hands wide open to receive it? Asking and being willing to receive are how your needs become your rising empowerment energy.

Brené Brown, best-selling author and shame researcher, talks about vulnerability a lot in her work and aptly describes it in her book *Daring Greatly*: "Vulnerability sounds like truth and feels like courage." It is a truth—an uncomfortable truth we have learned to keep hidden. That is why for some, being vulnerable takes a huge amount of courage, because when we allow others to see our softer, more emotional sides laid bare, we're exposed and open to attack. But if we do not lean into the mature expression of our needs—if we can't admit to, passionately ask for, and let in the things we want—nothing changes.

IT GETS MESSY

Here is the other big piece you should know up front: it's messy and emotional to do second-chakra healing work, and you can't skip over that. To get to the power of vulnerability, you have to meet your unmet needs where they started in the past. You have to go to the very vulnerable places that hold where you were hurt, disappointed, shamed, and even traumatized because of your needs. These are the places that can bring deep, meaningful healing.

Through the Healing Experience in this chapter, you will go through a radical process of undoing the coping mechanisms you put in place long ago. You'll get some revealing insight into why, when, and how you gave up your deepest needs and what your true needs are. Think of it as a fast track to finally figuring out what you really want in life or why you withhold pieces of yourself from others. Tapping and visualization will, step by step, take you through this messy process safely, compassionately, and at your own pace.

Most of us have learned to be extremely guarded around our soft sides and secret deepest needs, so expect some resistance and keep tapping. Follow your instincts on how many times you might need to tap through the scripts below, and stay with it, even if it takes weeks. This is important work and there is no rush.

HEALING EXPERIENCE #4: THE POWER OF VULNERABILITY

Setup Visualization #4-1

To get started take a deep breath. We are once again going to imagine that little inner child we tuned into in the first-chakra work. Children are wired to play. When they feel safe, a playful joy and imagination take over.

Take a deep breath and tune into your inner child. This time imagine the child is somewhere between the ages of three and six. If you are seeing a very young toddler, imagine they can speak to you clearly

See that little child in the place where you grew up at that age. First, just notice how the little one looks. Are they calm and happy or scared? Now imagine that you could step into that picture as the adult you are today and say the following to them:

I'm going to make it safe for you now, just you and me. I'm going to make it safe for you in this little space, just the two of us, for you to tell me what you really want. It is safe to tell me what you really want. What do you really want beyond safety? How do you want to be seen? How do you want to be treated? Do you want to be adored? Do you want everyone to listen and clap in amazement? Do you want to be the most amazing, the most special, or the most brilliant? What do you really want others to see in you?

Write down what your inner child says and note if it is extremely basic, such as *I just wanted to be safe/not get into trouble* or *I just wanted to be cared about.* If that is the message you are getting, really let that in and sit with it, and know that is extremely common.

Next, you are about to suggest something to this child that they are likely to disagree with, and I want you to listen to how they respond. Say to the child, *I want you to go and tell your parents right now what you really want. Go to your parents [or caregivers] and tell them what you just told me. Demand it.*

What does the child say? They will probably sound something like *No way. You don't understand. This will happen or that will happen. . . .*

Are they telling you that it's not even safe to ask because they will get in trouble? Are they telling you that it's impossible—that no one can meet that need? Are they telling you that they will be told that it's bad, maybe even by a look, or that it's inappropriate or shameful somehow? Do they feel guilty or bad for asking? Write down what your inner child is telling you, because this reaction is still what comes up in you when you ask for a need to be met.

In this round of tapping, we are going to voice the fear and reality of the child as if we were speaking *for* the child.

Tapping Script #4-1

There is my little child – And they are saying things like this – No way – I am not going to ask for that – There's no way that's safe – No way – If I ask for that – Or act like I want that – Act that special – It will not be safe for me – I will get in trouble – Or worse – If anyone sees what I want that bad – It will not be safe for me – It will not be safe for me – And they'll make me feel bad – They'll make me feel guilty – They've made it clear what's okay to want – And how I should act – It's not safe for me – No way, no way – I refuse, I refuse, I refuse to ask for this.

I will never ask for this – I will take this need, this desire – And I will push it down so far with fear – That I forget about it – I refuse to want it – It's not even safe for me to feel it – If I feel how badly I want it, it will be so painful – Because it will never ever be met – And it will be shamed – Me wanting it is bad – The fact that I want it proves – There's something bad about me – Not acceptable – Not acceptable – I refuse to want this – I will never ask for it – Even though it's what I want the most – And I'll figure out a way to want other things instead – To be seen in other ways – That feels safer – I will never admit I want this – I'll stop feeling it – Because it's bad – And it will never be a need that I can get met – It's just not safe – I'm only a child, and I've already learned all of this – This is just how it is for me.

Take a breath.

Post-Tapping Visualization #4-1

Tune into that child again. You just voiced their fear of wanting something that is a natural need and want for a child at that age and one of many natural rising impulses. You have heard how strongly they already believe it is bad and will lead to punishment. Their refusal to ask for that need directly from the only people who can fulfill it shows you how they've coped. You may have also seen an energy of resignation that sounds like *This is just the way it is for me.*

Second-chakra energy contains all your deepest needs, which shift and expand as you grow. However, the needs you see at this developmental age beyond the basics of simply being safe and loved remain at the core of your adult needs.

Tune into the child now and see how they look after you have voiced that for them. Do they feel understood? Can they tell that you get it now? Ask them again what they really want, keeping in mind the magical, playful mind of a child who feels totally safe and loved. Note the undertones of feeling special and adored.

Now take a moment to look at that child from your adult eyes. Is it okay for that child to experience the natural rising of all sorts of impulses, desires, and needs that sound special, powerful, and magical? Notice how simple their needs are. Notice that what they want from their parents may be things that you do naturally for young children now in your adult life—but you didn't get those things. Notice if you are, as an adult, adoring of children in your life, giving them attention and love and hugs and understanding, and clapping for them and saying, "You're amazing!" Maybe you as a little child did not get this, whether it was because it was not safe, there was just too much happening, it was a different generation where children were "seen and not heard," or there were rules about what was good or bad or "too much."

But now get clear within. Does this child, or any child, have the right to experience their natural need, want, and desire not only for love but to feel special, powerful, and adored? Is it wrong for a child to experience those feelings? Should they put them away? Feel guilty? Feel bad? Never feel them? Consider that these are likely many of the things you don't allow yourself to receive.

Take a breath and come back to the image in your mind's eye of the little child. Let's do a little bit of tapping and voice what we see and are holding a space for now.

Tapping Script #4-2

There's my little child – That was me – And there were things that I wanted – That I stopped asking for – Maybe even vowed – To never really want – To refuse to want – Because it wasn't acceptable or it wasn't safe – I would have been criticized or worse – But those things that I really wanted – Are things that a child is supposed to want – My impulse to not only be safe but loved – Not only taken care of but hugged and held – But to also be heard and seen – Seen for the real me – Really seen for the me I wanted to be even at that age – I had real needs – To be powerful even at that age – To be free enough to imagine and play – To be special in the eyes of my parents – Yes, to be adored for my specialness – Not for achieving anything – Just for being my childlike self – By shining as an innocent child.

But I learned to take those desires and those wants – And hold them back – Put them away – And I forgot about them – I lost them in the dark closet – I learned to fear them – And to judge them – And I locked them away – Like a side of me that was "too much" or "too weak" – Had to be locked away – A side of me that was always being let down – Had to be locked away.

But in my second chakra – Even today those are the things I want the most – And for my little child – I can see now that it wasn't fair – It wasn't fair, it wasn't fair, it wasn't fair – So much that child wanted – So much energy that wanted to flow up through me – Leading me forward – With joyfulness – And desires and wants – And I had to squeeze it down – Push it down – Contain it – The blasting energy of wants and desires – And impulses for joy, and fun, and play, and love – In the way that I wanted it – I had to contain it – To hold it tight, to hide it – And it wasn't fair, wasn't fair – I deserve better – I always deserved better – And I honor that now.

Take a breath and notice whether you are feeling sadness for the child and yourself.

If you were to picture yourself as that small child weeping alone, how would that feel in your heart? There are two reasons it is important to comprehend what you really did lose. First, to open second chakra energy, you must hear and honor grief. Honoring grief always opens up a very soft, vulnerable part of us. Second, it is likely that you are still denying yourself in your life right now, and it's costing you. What is the grief showing you? What are you still not allowing yourself to have?

Tapping Script #4-3

The truth is – I lost so much because of this – That little child that was me – Has been trapped inside me – Crying alone – And I honor that now – All those tears that had nowhere to go – No one to understand No safe arms to crawl into – No way to let them out – I try to be strong – And not want so many things – But there is a soft, vulnerable side of me – That has a deep well of sobbing tears – And that is hard to be with – But I want this grief to move – To let go of all these uncried tears – For everything I never got to have.

And I am open to hearing – The important messages in this grief – Of what I wanted – And what I still want – I honor all this sadness – All this loss – Everything I never got to have – And how much that has cost me – And may be still costing me – I would never let a child sob alone – So I honor this inner child of my second chakra – No more holding it in – No more pretending I don't need anything – No more locking my tears away in aloneness – I open my heart to myself – And give myself the compassion – And unconditional witnessing – Of love and understanding – That I need to heal my second chakra.

Take a deep breath and check in with yourself. If that tapping round was extremely emotional, you may want to break for today and come back to the next part tomorrow. Tuning into yourself and what you really need in this moment instead of blasting through the work is, in and of itself, second-chakra work.

Post-Tapping Visualization #4-3

Visualize this little child again. Let your mind paint a clear picture. Now that you've totally honored this child, you may see them as having shifted to a happier place. People are often surprised to see how quickly the child has moved into running off to play.

Let's build on that play for a minute and move energy in a different way. Close your eyes and see this child's second-chakra energy by imagining a small, brilliant, reddish-orange flame that starts just below their belly button and rises through their body. Someday that flame will include adult sexual energy, but right now it contains mostly needs and desires for physical safety, love, and affection; the calming, soothing feeling of being held; and the rising charge of playfulness and fun—running and falling, jumping, playing with friends, and rolling in the grass.

A special side of that charge is the rising natural impulse to be seen and experienced as special because you are *you.* Tune into that exuberant bursting energy of *Look at me! Listen to me! Look at me! Listen to me! Experience me as I'm experiencing myself!* See that energy flowing up through that child. So much energy. Let it be there full-on. Let yourself see this second-chakra energy free of fear of disappointment or a shaming or otherwise punishing reaction.

See that child aflame and just marvel at their beautiful, radiant, brilliant energy. Now give the child permission to grow into whatever they want to become, as big as they want to become, and with whatever powers they want to have. Watch as they transform into something that is magical or archetypal or an animal. Just let them grow with that big energy and notice everything about them. Notice the seeds of your adult gifts or just how big their energy is. (Couldn't you use some of that big energy sometimes?)

Your thinking mind has very little energy, and it's not the mind's job to have energy! Ideas alone can't power your life. The microprocessor that is your brain cannot power your life. You have to plug a computer into a power source to make it work. At the second chakra, you're looking at your power source—this is your battery pack, your inexhaustible power supply.

This is the empowerment energy that comes from your second-chakra desires, the caldron where your passion is created. It's very, very different than the joy we can experience in the upper chakras, which is more of an enlightened spiritual state. It's playful, sensual, powerful *Yes!* energy. This is where we ask not just with words but with our bold, passionate, enthusiastic energy and actions. And it is where we allow ourselves to receive. When what we want is offered, we readily say, *Yes, please, and thank you.* We ask and say yes with our second-chakra energy.

Now ask if your child is willing to share that energy with you by stepping into your body with that big reddish-orange flame of energy. Imagine that happening and notice how good it feels. This final round of tapping is something you can use again and again to reaffirm and even electrify your second-chakra energy.

Tapping Script #4-4

I don't have time for fear anymore – I don't have time for shame – I don't have time to be shut down with fear or shame about my second chakra – Because it's big – My second-chakra energy is a party of passion – And a Yes! *of desire and playfulness – It's a party of anger and rage sometimes – It's a fire hose of feeling myself – And what I really want – And feeling my passion – My power – And my softness, my vulnerability – I don't have time for guilt – I don't have time to be limited by the fear or shame I was taught as a child – Shutting down my desires to be special.*

Of course I want to be special – My desire to be seen and adored for who I am – Of course I want that – My desire to feel powerful – My own power shining – Of course I want that – My desire to be open and receive, receive, receive – Of course I want to receive – I love receiving – My desire to have sensual touch – And experience the world through my aliveness – That feeds me – I want this aliveness that blasts through – All of my desires – I am so alive.

In my second-chakra desires is where I remember that – I am so alive – And I want more *– I honor my second chakra – I probably have a lot more work to do – That's okay – I honor my second chakra – I need my second chakra – I need it for my mission – I need it to be powerful – I need it to enjoy every step – I need it to receive – And let things in – I even need it to make more money – And I definitely need it to have more fun – I honor my second chakra – And the rising, powerful energy it brings me.*

Take a breath and notice how you feel after this charged-up round of tapping. Do you suddenly feel like dancing or moving or going outside? That is quite common, and I highly recommend following that impulse to feel more second-chakra fun and energy. Notice how these feelings or impulses to move have an upward flow lifting you into action.

NEXT STEPS . . .

Be good to yourself and take it easy! Think of this as the beginning of a new relationship with a side of you that holds all your needs but may still have more tears to shed. As this side of you is heard, loved, and met with compassion instead of harsh words, it will reward you with a deeper knowledge of yourself and a deeper experience of joy. This is your second-chakra energy. It can lead the way to actually asking for and getting important things that you have always wanted—things that are often beneath our stated goals and efforts. But it is also a treasure chest of happiness, joy, childlike silliness, and energized drive!

Try to be a little less useful and a little more laughingly childlike for a few days. See how that feels and how the people around you react. Next, try asking the loving people in your life for what you need—such as a hug, a compliment, or loving attention—and see what happens.

Visit www.unblockedbook.com/chapter6 for an extra tapping experience and discussion to enhance this chapter.

CHAPTER 7

THE POWER OF ANGER

"Nope, you can't skip this part!"

"But, Margaret, I don't want to be angry! I am not an angry person."

I hear this all the time from people who are committed to personal growth and spirituality. In particular, I hear it from people who had an angry parent and have consciously vowed to "never be like that."

First, I promise this Healing Experience will not make you an angry, mean, or callous person. It will not turn you into anything like a parent or anyone else who used anger immaturely or as a weapon. Like the vulnerability work, the second chakra work around anger is counterintuitive and messy but important. It is another key to your treasure box of empowerment energy.

Through this Healing Experience, you will learn how to safely make contact with old spaces of reactionary anger and allow it to be voiced, honored, and moved so no one gets hurt, including you. This accomplishes two goals: First, it's critical for relearning how anger is supposed to move. Second, it frees you to experience the power and clarity it leaves behind. Transforming reactionary anger into empowerment energy is the key. This is the shift into courage and certainty of our rights and deserving that fills us with the fuel for self-preservation, assertiveness, advocacy, and the power to act.

After tapping you'll experience a new courage and authority when it comes to responding to unfairness. When the energy of anger and rage is safely (and maturely) moved, you have the courage to boldly go for what you want and say no to what you don't want. The gift is in having and allowing the energy of anger—which always gets triggered by something feeling unfair—to be used as a positive force.

Anger is intricately interwoven with your feelings of value and rights. The angry voice that says *It's not fair!* always leads to *And I deserve better!* So this voice holds a higher energy of honoring the self in many different ways—fair treatment, fair pay, or attention; the right to be happy, confident, and thriving; the right to go for what we want; and the right to be heard.

Anger is a big, rising energy. When it blasts through the nervous system as empowerment, you are suddenly able to push back, set a boundary, be louder, demand justice, and say no without that impulse being crushed by shame and insecurity. The rising energy of anger can overcome old habits and behaviors driven by guilt, fear, and shame and propel you into putting your foot down and making real changes in your life for the highest good.

You need your anger and even your rage energy to establish boundaries and declare "I deserve!" with 100 percent commitment. And you need it to fuel your passion. It takes work to build a business. It takes work to raise a family. It takes work to get a degree. It takes work to inspire social justice. And that means energy. You need this energy. It's kick-ass energy!

HEALING EXPERIENCE #5: THE POWER OF ANGER

Setup Visualization #5-1

Take a deep breath, close your eyes, and imagine that in your mind's eye you see a movie screen. The short flick that is about to play features someone who is angrily wronging or attacking you. The event could be recent or something that happened long ago. It doesn't matter how you're connected to this person. They could be a parent, an ex, a business partner—anyone who wronged you. Allow your mind to paint that picture. See this person standing there doing what they did and see yourself standing there too. This person really screwed you over. They wounded and betrayed you. Maybe they were openly angry and hostile, or maybe they thinly hid their anger in criticism, threats, or shaming.

See yourself in that situation with that person and notice how you reacted to being wronged. Maybe you were shocked and caught off balance, so you froze and didn't stand up for yourself. Maybe you broke down or let your anger loose. Or maybe you tried to calmly be diplomatic or people-please your way out of the situation. Notice you may have feelings about that. That's okay. Now imagine that something very strange happens, like a scene right out of an X-Men movie.

Imagine that a small child steps out of your body and stands next to you in the picture. But this is no ordinary child! It's the version of your second-chakra inner child that appeared in the last visualization as a magical or archetypal animal. But this time it is transformed by reactionary rage and fire into something powerful and dangerous. It is pure rage, and it is very angry at the person wronging you. Notice how it looks. This is your reactionary rage that has always been there for you anytime you have been wronged, disempowered, manipulated, guilted, shamed, or held back in any way. Whether you have ever shown it, felt it, or acknowledged it, this is part of you, and it gets enraged for you.

Look at that wild piece of you and see that as a child it is unconscious and primal in its "eye for an eye" rage. Now imagine it opens its mouth wide and starts yelling in protest.

Don't you push me. Do not try to intimidate me. Don't you take from me. Do not withhold from me what I deserve. Do not try to manipulate me. Step back or else! Notice what else it might want to say and imagine that and more.

What happens in that child-creature when it uses those words? How does the child look? See the flame of rage grow with massive, destructive power. Notice the quality of this rising energy that is coming to protect and advocate for you.

Let's tap to honor this primitive, reacting-to-unfairness rage energy.

Depression and Anxiety: Blocked Anger

Depression can happen when anger, over time, builds into frustration with no real outlet. The anger sits in our system. We're caged with it. After a while the repeated excruciating experience of stifling this empowerment energy becomes too much. We depress our anger as if to say, *It's not even worth it to get mad anymore. Nothing changes, so what is the point?*

Many clients who tell me they have had bouts of depression in their lives have a huge inner well of rage that has never been allowed to be expressed in a healthy way. Whenever they have gotten angry, it has led to something traumatic, shameful, or a relationship rupture that only reinforced their brokenness. These are often the same people who talk about suffering with anxiety or stress. This type of anxiety is the result of always trying to contain, not feel, and "get over" the massive amount of anger that they don't know how to move. In this case second-chakra tapping to voice and move the energy of anger is a truly life-altering process of going from resigned and stuck to energized and empowered.

Tapping Script #5-1

There it is, in all of its terrifying power – It is pure rage – Reactionary rage and anger – It is dangerous – And it does live in me – It lives in me – It is a volcano of rage – It is scary – This is the part of me that would fight to the death – If I needed to – So much power and energy – Terrifying – This part of me is terrifying – It looks like murderous rage consumed with anger and rage – Triggered by this person wronging me – It is so angry – There it is – And it feels totally justified – In its anger – It hates how this person is treating me – And it is ready and wanting to fight back – Push back – To stand up for me – So I can stand my ground – Because I am being wronged – Egregiously wronged – Unfairly wronged – And I totally honor that.

Note how strange it is to honor the protective motivation in your anger. We spend a lot of time not honoring our anger. Instead, we blame ourselves for things that happened to us. Blaming is really the opposite of honoring. It's telling ourselves, *I don't deserve to get angry because I brought this on myself.* Even lashing out in anger is not the same as intentionally hearing and honoring the hurt and unfairness. So look at the situation again, regardless of any mistakes you may have made, and ask yourself, *Did I deserve this?*

Tapping Script #5-2

It is strange to honor this rage-filled side of me – I am still against anger and rage – Because I know how badly it can be used – I know the pain of anger and rage – That turns into attacking and cruelty – And I honor that the dark side of anger is real – It is real in people – It is real in the world – But I also honor what I am seeing here – This part of me that is angry for me – And stands for me – And with me – Out of righteousness – Because I was wronged – That is true – And it really hurt – And I really did and do hate *that it happened – So I will stare into the face of my anger – This side of me that is unwavering – That is not afraid at all – And is* not *able to be manipulated – It will not back down to threats – Or be shamed – Or put in its place by guilt – It is impervious to guilt – Fearless and certain – It is raw courage – It is 100 percent certain that this is wrong – And that I don't deserve this bad treatment – It is solidly certain that I deserve better – And it is my fierce advocate – It arises to protect me – Advocate for me – Wanting to push back, hit back – For me – In defense of me – And what I deserve – Standing up for my rights – This is the voice of fearlessness – The energy of courage and readiness to fight – To take a stand – Right the wrong – The raw, terrifying power within me – I totally honor it – Yes, it can do horrible, terrible things – Maybe I hurt people with it in the past – Or have been hurt by the unchecked rage of others – In the shadows – It could be a monster – Sometimes this part turns on me – Attacks me – In the shadows – It is unconscious and it could be incredibly dangerous – And right now – I am just seeing it – Taking it in – And honoring it.*

Take a breath and check in with how you feel. Notice any emotion coming up or other bodily sensations and be with that, or tap without words if you need to.

Post-Tapping Visualization #5-2

See this part of you again as raw rage and do something that will seem even stranger. See the offending party again standing with you in the picture and let this wild creature side of you do whatever it wants to that person. On the movie screen of your mind, allow the wild creature to play out its terrible rage on that person. Keep watching until it is done. Note what it does. It is common to see this side of you fly into violent battle, killing with its hands or firing weapons much like in an archetypal battle in a computer-animated movie.

Now that the battle is over, notice how this part of you looks and feels. It will be in a calmer state. While your rage creature is in this calmer state, let it be filled with light. Fill it now with the light of consciousness.

See the real power and gift of the side of you that is always trying to come up and remind you about what you do and don't deserve. See the advocate in you that notices and reacts when someone acts like neither you nor your rights matter.

Anger is usually misunderstood and therefore not tolerated. But by not feeling and moving our anger, we squash this important voice and rising energy of courage. Notice that this side of you does not disappear. It remains in you, calm and strong and ready. What if, when you needed courage and clarity, you could harness this side of you when it was at a 2 instead of a 10 so you could speak your truth with the powerful energy of certainty?

If the wild one has been pent up for years, it will be reactive. But the more backlog of energy that is moved and honored, the more your anger will surface as a conscious voice and not a raging creature.

What is it that you really deserve that maybe you've been afraid to have? What is it that you really deserve but have felt too guilty to ask for? What do you really want and deserve?

For a minute bring back the bad person, the perpetrator. Put them once again into the picture with you. Notice how important they seem to you now. If the situation was traumatic, you may still have some more specific tapping to do around that person. But see if it now feels right to dismiss them as just not as important to you anymore.

What is important now is what you want. What do you really want instead of what you got in that scenario? What do you want from others and how do you want to be treated? What do you really want in life and how do you want to show up?

Close your eyes again and imagine that the calmer version of the rage creature steps back into your body and maintains its big energy. When there are no battles to fight, this is the energy of drive, passion, creation, and mission.

Tap and Rant

If you're upset with somebody, before you go into a conversation with them, tap and rant. That's my term for taking some time to tap through all the points using a script of your own making that gets at the heart of the problem. Complain, lambast, and lash out at the person until you're able to say exactly what it is that's making your blood boil (that is, what you really want), and you will feel calmer. Through tapping and ranting, you'll know what exactly is so upsetting to you (it's not always obvious) and can then approach any interaction with a mature energy that gets results.

Now that you are more conscious of your wild creature, be curious about this part of you. As you come to know and understand this energy, allow it to stay and pump through your system for creation, clarity, and courage. Let this piece of energy rise through your system into your voice and notice whether you're able to speak more honestly than maybe you ever have about what you want and how much you want it.

I invite you to want things as if going another day without them would be awful, painful, and leave you feeling half alive! That's what it means to feel alive and passionate.

This next tapping script is designed to encourage rising empowerment energy and build up a charge. Fill in the blanks with things you really want. And don't hold back!

Tapping Script #5-3

The truth is – There are so many things I want – Things I really want – And have been hoping for – And waiting for – And I am kind of sick of not having them – Sick of waiting – And I am really sick and tired of people wronging me – I don't want that anymore – I don't want to attract that anymore – I don't want to be in battle anymore – I want to be free to create my life – I totally deserve that – I am not perfect, but I definitely deserve that – I want people who are awesome and honest – And conscious in my life – I want to feel alive – And go for what I really want – I want to feel my confidence – And feel courage when I need it – And I really want to have more fun too – And I want very specific things – I want ____________ . I want ____________. I want ____________. Oh, and I would also really love *___________! – And I am now declaring – That when those things and people and opportunities show up – I will say* yes to them *– I will happily say,* Yes, thank you! *– When they show up – I won't wonder if I deserve them – Or feel guilty –* No way *– I will say a big yes to all these things showing up in my life – For my highest good – Yes to receiving – Yes to asking for more – Yes to more joy and passion – Yes to more fun – Yes to more compliments, friends, and good times – Yes to more brilliance – Yes to bold action – Yes to me and my deserving – Yes to all of me – Watch out world – Here I come!*

ON THE OTHER SIDE OF ANGER

When you honor and safely voice anger, you come out of anger on another side. You move from rage to outrage to courage, the most mature expression of anger. Courageous action inspires win-win outcomes. It brings people together. It fuels meaningful change. And it feels good. We know that's what is on the other side.

We carry real pain from being around reactive, hurtful anger, but we need to start separating our reactive anger from the message in it by shifting into this reverence. Anger that has been unable to move you into empowerment can build up like a volcano that needs to be handled properly, like a child who's having a big tantrum.

Transforming anger can happen in a matter of minutes, which is why tapping is the most miraculous tool. You can move from the pure unconscious rage of anger and unfairness into the less reactive and more mature clarity and certainty about what you really want. In this way you'll often find that whatever was pissing you off before either no longer matters or sets you on your empowered, positive mission.

Your second-chakra rage is power. It's a huge piece of your power, and it needs to be handled and beheld with the utmost reverence. It's tricky because it's such a scary animal. It can be used so badly. It can cause so much pain and suffering in the world, and it does! It causes pain and suffering in our relationships and our families.

NEXT STEPS . . .

This week stop and tap on anger at least once per day. Go ahead and sound over-the-top angry, even if you just feel a little annoyed. Really lean into it. Do it in your car or in a safe place where no one will hear you, but voice whatever you are angry, frustrated, disappointed, or annoyed about *very, very loudly.* Don't try to fix it or be positive. Just let your anger, hate, or resentment speak unchecked as you tap. Then when you feel calmer, ask yourself these important questions: *What do I really want instead? And how bad do I want it?*

Visit www.unblockedbook.com/chapter7 for an extra tapping experience and discussion to enhance this chapter.

CHAPTER 8

THE POWER OF LIFE-FORCE ENERGY

Raw life-force energy is another term for survival energy. We're born with this energy that causes us to kick and scream and cry. As we grow up, this inborn survival energy shifts from ensuring survival to powering our drive and vitality, moving us to create, manifest, learn, and follow a passion.

In this Healing Experience, we're going move into the energy of sensuality and sexuality, your largest channel of raw life-force energy. Sexual energy flows not just for sexual activity but for all creative sparks. It's the energy of attracting and manifesting what you truly desire, together with the energy of being open to receiving that manifestation.

Author Caroline Myss talks about how the sexual energy channel is intricately connected to how we create and manage money and wealth in our lives. So when you work on this aspect of your second chakra, you'll also experience a new charge in how you sensually experience and enjoy your work; a new spark in creativity, energy, and delicious fun; and, if you choose, a deepening of your ability to be sexually intimate in your relationship.

Don't worry. This Healing Experience isn't just for the young or partnered. Even if you are not in a relationship or if you think of yourself as "not needing that anymore," you benefit from uncovering and clearing all the blocks and beliefs keeping you from honoring the powerful fire hose that is your sexual energy channel.

Also, this work is not going to take you into the dark side of sexuality. This is not about caricatures or extremes. It is about owning your magnetic, compelling, charismatic energy. So again, don't worry.

This work is for *you and only you* first. It is a pathway to loving and adoring and rejoicing in more parts of yourself more deeply than you ever have. Take a moment to think about that. This work is about how you feel about you and your many types of power, not just your power to think intellectually or your power for self-discipline and hard work. It is about feeling and appreciating your compelling, charming, magnetic power—the joyful, playful radiance in you that naturally draws in people, opportunities, resources, support, and more. This work will make you seem luckier because things will start to line up for you with ease.

This work is also about vibrant health! Life-force energy is an rising energy of vitality and rejuvenation. Think of how alive and present and amazing we feel when we fall in love. No matter the age, people will always say they "feel young again," and that just feels good. It doesn't feel good to push it down.

Your seductive and pleasure-seeking side holds such vitality and power and opens so many doors that it's essential to build a solid relationship with and understanding of it. The payoff is huge when it comes to feeling more alive, more powerful, and having a more magnetic, compelling energy around other people without being "overtly" sexual. It can also trigger a reconnection to sexuality that you can explore in your intimate relationship with yourself and your partner.

A History of Sexual Trauma

Those of you with a history of sexual trauma may find tapping through the scripts in this section incredibly triggering. This may not be a section to work through on your own. This process in particular may trigger past trauma that needs to be addressed with the proper space and support for healing.

Tapping is a proven-effective trauma-healing technique and has been used gently and successfully for many years with people who suffer from PTSD. But if you have a history of sexual trauma, it will still likely be a challenge to open this energy channel by yourself because it won't feel safe. Be kind to yourself, know your limitations, and proceed with care and the right support.

HEALING EXPERIENCE #6: THE POWER OF LIFE-FORCE ENERGY

Setup Visualization #6-1

In this Healing Experience, we will be tuning into your body again, but this time we'll go beyond body acceptance into rejoicing in our body. We will use the word *sexy* because it is charged, filled with meaning, and will reveal any resistance and fears about holding this specific type of energy. It allows you to challenge self-perceptions of your power, your worthiness, and the limitations on how good you can feel about yourself. Feeling sexy goes beyond just feeling good about yourself or how you look on any given day. In the feminine energy, feeling sexy is feeling like a goddess-warrior. In the masculine energy, it's the pure swagger of the hero.

Start by taking a deep breath. See yourself standing there in front of that mirror we used in our first chakra work, only this time you're wearing a bathing suit. Yes, it's bathing-suit season! No hiding in your clothes.

See yourself standing in front of the mirror in your bathing suit and look at your body closely. Now say out loud, "I'm sexy and powerful." Then measure on a scale of 1 to 10 how true that feels where 1 is not true at all and 10 is completely true. And notice if you're already tuning in to some really specific physical things about your body that are preventing you from feeling sexy.

In the following tapping script, the words are pretty negative. If you are one of the people for whom these words do *not* resonate and you easily love and honor your sexiness, then you may not need this part of the work at all. Or you can change the words to match how you feel. If this is already hard for you, substitute any words or criticisms or specific body parts that are loud in your head.

Tapping Script #6-1

There I am – I am so not sexy – Ohh, noo – I am not sexy at all – I don't deserve to feel sexy – Look at me – Look at that body – Maybe I accept it a little more now – But it's not sexy – Sexy means something different – Sexy means perfect – And that's not me – I refuse to feel sexy – It's not right – It's not safe – Because of my body, I refuse to feel sexy – I can't, even if I wanted to – And society would agree with me.

This is not a sexy body in front of me – I am so not *sexy – Look at all the things wrong with my body – Maybe I'm lovable – But with this body, I can't be sexy – I can't pull that off – I'm not going to let myself feel that – Feel that energy – Feel that flow of power – It's dangerous – It's inappropriate – Maybe it's a long-gone part of my life – And I have really good reasons – I'm gross! – Embarrassing – Not perfect – Parts are so ugly – Not sexy at all.*

If I were to try to act sexy – That would be a joke – I refuse to let myself feel the fun, energetic feeling of sexy – I refuse to feel that big energy – That red-carpet, fabulous energy – That's not for me – And the truth is – It doesn't even feel safe to talk about it.

Take a deep breath.

Again, the second chakra is where your most vital aliveness energy flows up through your system—your passion, your desire, your needs, and your "yes to receiving" energy that balances all your "doing" energy. A big piece of that channel is "energetically attractive" and magnetic. It draws in hero swagger or goddess-warrior energy and goes way beyond sexuality.

This is the point where you may start to feel unsafe in this process if you have wounding around your sexuality. So this next round will voice a range of fears that will have an intensity unique to you. If it feels overwhelming, let go of the words and just keep tapping and breathing. Work this whole process slowly. Take a break and get support if you need it.

Let's tap through the points again.

Tapping Script #6-2

I'm really feeling this – I'm really feeling the resistance to it – Even starting to feel sexy is triggering some resistance – If I let myself feel sexy, I do believe bad things will happen – I am very afraid I will attract something bad – Maybe that happened before – And that means there will be pain and ugliness – Humiliation or physical attack – Or that I will be used – Or maybe ridiculed and rejected – Feeling good about myself – Too good – Will lead to something very scary – Dangerous – Out of control – Out of my control – And I made a vow to never let that happen – To never be vulnerable like that – To never carry power like this – This attractive power – This attractive goddess energy.

Because it will attract something negative – Something painful, something shameful – I'm really feeling this resistance – It's dark – It's yucky – It's stuck in my second chakra – This vow to never use my powerful, magnetic, attractive energy – To not let people see it – To not use my pulling, receiving, and allowing power – Because it would make me too vulnerable – I learned to squelch and disown – My compelling, charismatic, energetic power that is my sexy feeling – It's not safe – It's really scary, and I've attached so many beliefs to this – That I learned in painful, scary moments – So many judgments about my body – So many judgments about when I can be sexy – And when I can't – And society agrees with me.

So many good reasons to not feel sexy – To not allow this energy – I won't do it – I won't do it – I refuse – I'm just going to honor that – I've put a lid on a volcano in my second chakra – The volcano of my life-force energy – I've put a cork in it – It's still there, but the volcano is real – And I'm just going to honor that too.

I'm open to healing all of these wounds at my second chakra – Little by little – It is my intention to take baby steps to heal – This entire part of my body – That's been carrying these wounds and vows for me – I'm so open to healing it – Not sure yet what that will mean in my life – And baby steps mean I can figure it out slowly – But I'm so open to healing it – I totally honor my second chakra – My sexuality – And my power.

Take a deep breath and notice where you are emotionally. Be ready to tap through that script multiple times if the negative words still feel true. When you tap through the script again, this time read the words without speaking them out loud. Focus in on all the feelings and sensations in your body. If you feel nauseated or shaky or weird, get up and move! Shake your body like a dog shakes off water, stamp your feet on the floor to help ground yourself, scream into a pillow or pound your fists on some thick cushions or your bed. Physical movement will help release stuck second-charka energy.

Post-Tapping Visualization #6-2

Once you are ready to move on, close your eyes and tune into the mirror again. See yourself there in your bathing suit and again say, "I am sexy and powerful!" Check in with how true that feels now on scale of 1 to 10 where 1 is not true at all and 10 is completely true. After enough tapping your number should be higher. Do you feel a little sexier? A little less vulnerable around being sexy? Are you less negative about your body?

Note whether you are now noticing something specific about your body that you don't like that is keeping you stuck. It might sound something like *I can't be sexy because of my* ________ (fill in the blank). You can keep working on that very specific thing by tapping through the points again. Just keep repeating that sentence and adding in any other criticism or judgment you have about that part of your body.

After you start to feel calmer, tune into the mirror again, but now imagine you have changed into your favorite (or favorite type of) outfit. Let it be something that you easily feel fabulous, hot, and sexy in—something that makes you feel like you love your bad self. Maybe it's a dress, sportswear, a leather coat, or a tailored suit. Now take it up a notch by imagining yourself strutting across the room or twirling and then stopping for a pose. Hold that image, and let's do more tapping.

Tapping Script #6-3

There I am – I totally honor that I'm more than medium – That I'm pretty fabulous – That I am sexy in my way – And that the truth is – Feeling sexy is a feeling that rises up on the inside – Lots of different people – With lots of different body shapes – Feel sexy out there – Some of them are role models – So I'm just going to let myself feel totally sexy.

Just for me right now – For me alone – Fabulous, red-carpet sexy – I love that feeling – It's fun, it's silly, it's playful, it's kind of awesome – Powerful, attracting, sexy – I'm open to feeling that massive flow of energy – Owning my inner goddess or my smoldering swagger – Confident and strutting – Just for a minute, letting myself feel it – Feel really awesome – *The pure, sensual sensation of feeling so good and delicious in my skin – Loving my bad self – Sexy, awesome, fabulous – Standing on the red carpet – Oh, yeah – That's me.*

Take a deep breath.

If you still feel a lot of negativity or resistance, or too vulnerable, keep tapping to the previous scripts until this positive round feels good.

Post-Tapping Visualization #6-3

If you're just feeling sexy, I really want you to let yourself be with that and how playfully fun it is. Nothing else has changed in the outside world. Your body hasn't physically changed in the last few minutes, but suddenly you can bring up this feeling of being right there on the red carpet, fabulous and sexy.

Close your eyes again and look at yourself now in that mirror. Imagine that you can see your energy field around you. How does your energy look? Think of someone who carries their goddess or swagger energy in a beautiful way—someone whom you admire or an archetypal figure such as a Greek god or goddess who resonates with your kind of sexy. Bring them into that picture and imagine them merging into you, allowing you to inhabit that same flavor of second-chakra power. How do you look now, and how does that feel?

Think about what happens next. When you're feeling fabulous and sexy and standing there on the red carpet, think about your level of worthiness. How worthy do you feel? And how worthy do you feel asking for your needs to be met?

The second chakra is where we engage the Law of Attraction—a universal law that says we attract what we focus our energy and attention on. It's literally when we ask for something and it is given. This is different from the fifth, or Throat, chakra, where you ask with your voice. Manifesting requires asking with your second chakra—that vital, effortless attracting and receiving energy. When you feel your deepest needs—feel what you really want—you're already asking. And through that asking you open to receiving. It's putting your arms out to receive something versus having your arms crossed and saying, "I don't want anything."

That's second-chakra asking. When you allow yourself to feel that, you don't even have to open your mouth. Your second-chakra energy attracts and pulls toward you the people and events that make your dream a reality. So two balancing aspects of the second chakra are that you're expanding power and energy and feeling that, and you're expanding attracting, receiving, and asking energy.

Tune into that image of you in the mirror again and realize that you can be in this powerful second-chakra energy in any circumstance without acting overtly sexy or even with no sexual energy at all. What would happen if you walked into any room—even a business meeting—and inside, you had this energy of *Yeah. That's right. I'm powerful.* It's a totally fabulous energy. It's charisma. It's self-love in the most beautiful way, and it's *very* attractive, compelling, and persuasive. It's your very own rock-star quality!

NEXT STEPS . . .

Your assignment this week is to make this commitment to yourself: *I'm going to take a baby step in practicing what it is like to see and feel myself as powerful, fabulous, and sexy.* You can practice this completely alone. Just take a few minutes to put on a song you love and strut around your house like a model or a rock star. This should feel fun, ridiculous, silly, and maybe even a little embarrassing, even though no one's watching. That is okay! Keep playing with it!

Do you notice any difference in how things appear after doing this exercise? When you feel sexy, powerful, and valuable, everything around you feels more alive and fabulous. It's like falling in love but with yourself. The second chakra has the key to opening your heart to your beauty, and this allows you to see—to behold—more beauty and radiance in everything and everyone.

Visit www.unblockedbook.com/chapter8 for an extra tapping experience and discussion to enhance this chapter.

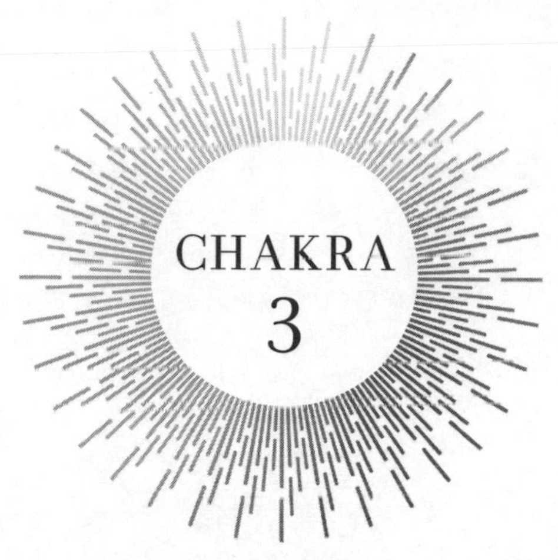

THE POWER TO ACT—HEALING THE SOLAR PLEXUS CHAKRA

Fear? What fear?
Shout "*Yes, I want this!*"
Rising energy, enthusiasm,
and courage will *lift* you
into *bold* action.
Hesitation is *so* last year!

CHAPTER 9

RECLAIMING CONFIDENCE AND ASSERTIVENESS

Imagine you're in a casino. In the corner is a slot machine with a large flashing neon sign: *$1 Slots. Win $2 Million!* Never before has the pot been that high. Imagine your building excitement and enthusiasm when you think that, by spending only one dollar, you could become a millionaire. You don't think twice before putting a dollar in the machine. What have you got to lose? When enthusiasm is high and the risk is low, we aren't conflicted about whether we should do something. We just act. It doesn't even take courage. We can't get our dollar out fast enough.

Now imagine you're back in the casino the next day. The one-armed bandit still offers a $2 million purse, but the price to play has gone up to $3,000. The risk just got higher. You might feel some butterflies and fear. You might just say forget it and walk away. It's the same game you were more than eager to play the day before, but now that you have more to lose, even if the payoff is still high, it's a bit scary. You think twice before throwing in your chips.

What most people miss about the universal problems of inertia, procrastination, distraction, and self-sabotage is the level of risk. When we experience any of these problems, the risk of taking the action is too high for us. The first chakra is controlling the system. It's reminding us that if we do such-and-such, we won't be safe. It's the $3,000 bet. If we don't have enough energy in the bank—enough second-chakra enthusiasm, courage, or passion—to overcome the risk, we won't take the chance.

Now let's up the ante. In a third scenario, you have a 1-in-3 chance of winning, but to pull the lever, you have to get up in front of everyone and do a three-minute TED Talk on how gifted and passionate you are. Actor and comedian Jerry Seinfeld joked that at a funeral, most people would rather be in the casket than give the eulogy. That's how afraid most people are of public speaking—let alone praising themselves!

In this third scenario, the risk is extreme. You start to feel the fear—the first-chakra fight-flight-freeze-bond response—as if you are about to do something life-or-death. It's really hard to talk yourself out of this kind of fear. The conscious, logical mind is up against this long-forgotten but deeply held certainty that there is too much risk. Your nervous system kicks in, and you start to sweat and feel anxious. All you can think about is how vulnerable you'd feel. The audience might start throwing tomatoes, and you would be standing there completely exposed. Who are you to be praising yourself anyway—and for a full three minutes?

Because belonging is a primitive survival reality, the risk of being rejected can trigger life-or-death fear—survival fear. No way you are playing this game. You cash in your chips and step outside, where those feelings of anxiety dissipate and you feel safe again.

Characteristics of the Solar Plexus Chakra

Located in the pit of the stomach, in the center of the torso, the Solar Plexus Chakra is the seat of our hero energy. In action it looks and feels like the part of the novel or movie where the main character gathers the will to finally step up, take big action, and make a change for the better.

The third chakra is our action center. When third-chakra energy is flowing, we are primed to act and take charge to get what we want or make a difference. We call on the third chakra to push through potential risks and go for it. We exude self-esteem, a strong identity, and total respect for self. Our enthusiasm and will for action are on fire.

In the third chakra, we see how guilt shrinks power and how moving our emotions liberates the energy we need to take bigger action. Playing it small is not on the menu. The Sacral Chakra empowers us to act and speak with enthusiasm and present ourselves as valuable members of any tribe. It encourages us to be visible and noticeable—to lead with authority and risk exposing our true selves even in the face of criticism. Here, we revere ourselves as true and sacred *miracles,* called to make a difference in the unique way that only we can.

THREE CHAKRAS WORKING AS ONE

What separates risk-takers from those who play it safe? In my book risk-taking is not defined by the degree of actual danger but by how safe or unsafe *we feel* when taking the risk. The guy who gets up on a stage with only a two-foot-wide podium as a shield could be taking just as much risk as the guy who walks on a one-inch-wide wire across a live volcano.

There's a thin line between real-time and remembered danger—those old hot-stove moments. Our first chakra nervous system wiring has learned that exposing ourselves, or leaving ourselves wide open to criticism and rejection, can be just as life-threatening as walking over a live volcano, so we feel a blast of fear. Even public speaking, which is in most instances a safe and secure proposition, causes our bodies to react as if our very lives were at stake.

The first, second, and third chakras are interdependent. When a flowing first chakra tells us without a doubt that we are intrinsically deserving and have the right to pursue and have what we want, that second-chakra passion energy fills the third-chakra action center with the charge to push through the potential risks and *go for it*. Risk schmisk! We boldly go after what we want with our words and actions.

When a blocked first chakra is running the show—telling us the risk is too high and we will not be safe if we go there—second-chakra passions are stymied. Third-chakra energy, which is supposed to take those passions and run, has nowhere to go. It's bottled up. We stew with resentment or feel stuck or frustrated. We never get behind that podium, much less walk on a wire. We don't start that new diet plan, apply for that promotion, write that book, or take that dream vacation. Our days are flat and predictable. It's Groundhog Day again—just like in the movie.

ON A GUILT TRIP

When the fear of breaking tribal rules that we have learned at our first chakra arrives at our third chakra, it is called guilt. Guilt is a powerful and uncomfortable feeling that tells us what we are doing, thinking about doing, or have already tried to do is based in a bad or shameful intention. Guilt will shut down our third-chakra action center in a heartbeat, rendering us unable to do anything except succumb to patterns of behavior that that we've relied on in the past—backing down, walking away, hiding, isolating, or working harder to prove we're a team player and not a threat to anyone.

Half the time we don't realize guilt is a driving force because we scrupulously avoid doing or saying the things that would trigger it. So most of how we act, speak, and show up is driven by *avoiding* feeling guilty. We, for instance, don't submit those college applications because our parents expect us to take over the family business. We won't even suggest going on that cruise because our spouse would see it as foolishly spending resources. In either instance we'd be called out as being selfish. Following our natural impulses becomes an act of selfishness, which makes us feel guilty.

The risk of being exposed as selfish triggers guilt and trips most of us up. Many solopreneurs, for instance, can't even think of raising their prices or setting a boundary with a client who is always asking for more without paying more.

The only benefit to feeling guilty is that it ensures we feel safe. We are in our comfort zone, even if that zone is consistently unfair, draining, and disempowering.

STAYING IN OUR LANE

I like to describe the comfort zone as "staying in our lane" or "not rocking the boat." An exaggerated version of this is the managed way we might speak to a police officer when pulled over for speeding. We act differently than we normally would—partly out of fear and the weight of potential consequences. It's just more comfortable to play it safe.

The comfort zone is fine, even necessary, for periods of time. We hardly even notice we are in it. But life is not about staying static, safe, and in the same lane. It's about growth and potential. So at certain points in life, we will feel a second-chakra impulse to be more than we are and do something bold. This sometimes shows up in a dream or when we suddenly have an idea that sparks excitement. Based on these impulses, we start scheming about what we need to do to make this dream happen. And then we set some goals.

Goals that push us out of our comfort zone and require breaking the rules of the past or overstepping certain boundaries will eventually start to feel worrisome. We begin to focus on the expected negative reactions: *What if I get criticized? What if no one likes my ideas, or what if no one even cares? What if others judge me? What if people become jealous of my wealth or power and come after me, attack me, steal from me, or use me? Why should I spend the time and energy doing something that won't work out anyway?*

The nervous system, which we know is wired for safety, kicks in and slows us down with some variation of the fight-flight-freeze-bond response. In our modern times, we are likely to bond. This nervous-system reaction ensures that we act accordingly so that we still belong with our tribe members, even at the expense of self-respect. This can also be called the accommodate-and-cooperate response. We laugh along when someone insults us, for instance, or continue being a team player to someone who is actively wronging us. Remember that belonging is life. It's survival. Rejection is death.

The big fear is facing hostility or attack from members of our tribe. As we grow, we threaten the comfort zone of some—or even all—of our tribe members. They might even try to hold us back without being fully conscious of why they're doing it. Their goal is not necessarily to hurt us but to keep us in line—to ensure we respect tribal rules. But as we touched on in Chapter 5, tribes can change, and sometimes we have to let go of tribal members who aren't there for us—or at least let go of how much influence we'll allow them to have over us.

To step out of our comfort zone, we almost always need different people—a new set of tribe members who relate to our dreams and struggles and are happy to cheer us on. We most definitely need a different version of ourselves.

STEPPING OUT AND UP-LEVELING

To reach new heights, we need a bigger, bolder, stronger version of ourselves. We can find it by unblocking the third chakra, which has the energy burst we need to step outside our comfort zone. It starts with getting extremely clear on what our specific worrisome expectation is: What makes us stop in our tracks?

How do we do that when we are already stuck? In the Healing Experience chapters, we'll use a process called Healing Forward to visualize what would happen if we boldly stepped up. This reveals all the fears that prevent us from moving forward and how intense they are on a scale of 1 to 10. This is typically a huge aha moment for most people because for the first time they understand *why* they have been stuck and holding back.

Instead of beating themselves up for not taking action, people are suddenly compassionate with themselves because they actually see how high the risk is. Healing Forward also makes it possible to laser-focus healing efforts on the exact action we want and need to take.

This is important work because just the thought of getting out of our lane and standing out can create a lot of anxiety, and we only need a little anxiety to stop us. Take, for example, the person who spends years training for a certain skill set. They might achieve the highest level of certification but never market themselves. The person who has a story to tell might attend one writing seminar after another and read every book on the topic but never write their book. Or they might write it but won't do anything to market their creation. Others might set a health goal for eating better or exercising but lack the willpower to change their habits. They end up cheating on their own goals.

I ask my clients to view the process of looking at the deeper fears behind stepping out as a fascinating route of self-discovery, not just as something to fix. Each time we discover a new fear or insecurity that is the root of procrastination, for example, we learn more about ourselves, our needs, *and* exactly what to tap away to unblock third-chakra energy. This gives us that boost of enthusiastic *Yes!* energy. We start taking bolder action, and that kind of growth-in-action reveals a new level of fear. So we tap on it and release more fear of the unknown and unblock even more third-charka energy. Our life starts to change because we're finally changing lanes and moving forward in new, exciting ways.

This is up-leveling. Voicing, moving, and honoring a fear frees natural energy to rise and build. We feel challenged and compelled to become more of who we are. We up-level to new heights we couldn't even conceive of in our comfort zone. This process of growth, action, self-compassion, and self-discovery morphs us into that bigger, bolder, stronger version of ourselves. We can even become the hero of our own story.

Cost of a Weak Third Chakra

- Taking action seems like a no-win situation
- Feeling stuck all the time
- Fearing and avoiding stepping up and being seen or being the center of attention
- Overthinking instead of getting into action
- Running on anxiety
- Feeling shame or guilt whenever you try to self-advocate or ask for more
- Believing in and acting on a vow to self-sacrifice, always give, and never be selfish
- Anger getting stuck and becoming resentment
- Experiencing extreme difficulty saying no or setting boundaries, unless concrete external reasons justify or force it

Benefits of a Strong Third Chakra

- The massive energy of the second chakra flowing up to the third chakra, where you embody the true, powerful *you* and take action from your real power, desire, and needs
- Accessing a bolder, rock-star quality of charisma and presence whenever needed; dynamically bringing it up or pulling it back to match the circumstance
- Acting enthusiastically and willing to be seen and declare yourself as valuable
- Feeling a bigger charge of energy and action that is clear and focused on the most important things (even action you have avoided for years)

- Being able to stand in your truth, ask for what you want more boldly, and take action with passion and charisma to create your desires
- Feeling *delighted* in just being you
- Easily setting personal boundaries that honor you and others, without confrontation, battle, or trauma

A HERO'S JOURNEY

Earlier we talked about how the third chakra holds our hero energy. A great way to illustrate how blocked third-chakra energy finally moves is to talk about the classic hero's journey. Most movies carry a similar hero's journey theme: The main character starts at a place of status quo or hiding his power. We might judge him a little bit in that part of the movie, thinking he's weak or insignificant or foolish. Then some difficulties start to go down. This character gets bullied, attacked by some dark force, or challenged in some way. For a while he keeps taking a beating and does not fight back. He feels like a cowardly loser in a no-win situation. By the time we reach that point in the movie, compassion replaces judgment. We feel for the guy and want him to fight back and win!

Interestingly, when *we* are in that phase of *our* movie, we couldn't be more critical and judgmental. We look back at times in our life and a part of us says, *I should have been stronger. I shouldn't have been afraid. I should have been more courageous. I should have. I should have. I should have.*

In the movie the main character eventually gets angrier and angrier until all his rage blasts through his system, and he does what he needs to do at the third chakra. He puts his foot down and says, "That is it. No more. I don't care if I get beaten. I don't care if I'm afraid. This is so unfair. I am doing something different. I am going to stand up and fight. I'm going to push through my fear and whatever it is telling me I shouldn't do. I will not live this way any longer. I will not let this contain me."

His rage is a natural uprising against being wronged, and he is finally on a mission to free himself and possibly others from oppression. When we hear that outrage and feel the inherent sense of honor and leadership when he accepts the responsibility to take a stand and face the risk with courage, we cheer for him. "Finally!" we say as we feel the same rising energy in ourselves.

This pattern happens in real life. First, we take it, and we take it, and we take it. Then we start to get enraged or sad, and then we can't take it anymore. At this point one of two things happens: either we listen to the message that our outrage (our justified anger) is delivering, and we take action, or at the moment we most need our rage, we experience a power shortage—the collapsing, depressing force of shame.

"Mama Bear" Energy

Some people may be unwilling to get mad for themselves, but if they see other people—tribe members or those who are more vulnerable than them—getting hurt, they are suddenly moved into action. This is often where very sensitive or otherwise mellow people find their biggest power—their "mama bear" energy. They can take the pain themselves, but they can't stand to see another person, an animal, or even the environment being hurt or treated unfairly. "That's so wrong! She does not deserve that!" In advocating for someone or something else, empowerment energy moves us to action with certainty, courage, and strength.

JUSTIFIED ANGER

We've talked a lot about reactionary anger, or the in-the-moment nervous-system response to something that is simply not fair. As explosive as it can be, reactionary anger is always hiding a painful and scary hurt. It's reacting to some external event that feels cruel and unfair *without acknowledging the hurt or the unfairness.*

Everyone is familiar with anger that stews or feels more like frustration. But when we acknowledge the truth about an unfairness and its effect on us or others as well as the cost—and we know we did not deserve it—our anger will feel justified. Justified anger will rise as outrage as we get ready to protest. This is where we draw a line in the sand, speak up, set a boundary, and take action. Justified anger dispels guilt. Now we have the right to be angry because this is so unfair. Justified anger always has at its root compassion, either for ourselves or another. When expressed honestly, it comes out with a lot of deeply held or guarded hurt, which *is* the key to truly healing and releasing it.

The more honest response to an unfair situation is to say, "That really hurt. It's really unfair that I have to do your chore on top of everything else I do, and I'm hurt because you don't seem to recognize all I do." That's the real feeling we need to get to. Unfairness, then, is a tool we can use to get to the heart of an unmet need or whatever is causing the hurt.

Moving blocked third-chakra energy always requires facing unfairness with either justified anger or hurt. They are the only emotions that have enough energy to blast through and dispel third-chakra guilt, which in this case is saying it's wrong to speak up for ourselves.

POWER SHORTAGES

When we won't allow ourselves to feel either reactionary or justified anger, we experience a power shortage. Power shortages usually show up in the third chakra when we need our energy the most.

A common experience for many women in my generation, for example, is freezing up, laughing off an insult, and going along silently when a male boss or co-worker says or does something inappropriate or insulting. Later we wonder why we put up with it, why we didn't push back or act as outraged as we should have. Infuriated with ourselves for our lack of courage or quick thinking, we imagine all the things we could have said or done. We end up blaming ourselves, because we "could have" or "should have" done or said X, Y, or Z. Suddenly someone else's poor behavior is our fault. Families, businesses—much of society—have been quick to reinforce these self-inflicted feelings of idiocy, asking, "Why did you put up with that? Why didn't you just say no?"

A lifetime of habit around restricting the *Hey, I deserve better* energy that is anger means that instead of being filled with the energy, courage, and commanding voice that justified anger brings, we can only freeze and fall back on the submissive strategies we have learned. Accommodating and giving in are poor substitutes for setting clear boundaries, but they are default responses. In these cases we lose twice—once in the moment and again when blaming ourselves for our utterly confounding weakness.

Pushed-down anger keeps us stuck, and feeling stuck means being frustrated, disappointed, and resentful. Guilt ensures we stay stuck. People will agonize over decisions, even minor ones, for hours and sometimes years because they feel guilty about following a passion: *But I feel guilty, and then my family guilts me, and I don't know what to do. . . .* That kind of indecisiveness always involves a power shortage. We are refusing to own our power or set a boundary. Meanwhile we go through months or years of irritation and seething resentment while smiling and continuing to do something we don't want to do. The lack of decisiveness that comes from not being able to own our power because our anger is stuck wastes massive amounts of time and energy.

Another form of power shortage comes from lack of feeling. If we can't feel, we can't desire. When we don't desire, the aliveness and inner joy that comes from being truly fulfilled is missing. If asked, we wouldn't be able to say what it is we really want in life. We keep trying to "figure it out" with lots of thinking, but we never get too far.

Occasionally we might get clear about a passion building inside and feel a surge of energy to dive in and make a big change. But instead of following through on big ideas and exciting plans, we get stuck, procrastinate, and spin our wheels. The moment of passion that may have kick-started a new path fades just as it is needed most. This restriction can go on for years in some, days in others, until impulses and strong feelings unexpectedly build and explode.

HOW CHANGE HAPPENS

It all comes back to what we learned as a child. If we learned from an explosive parent that all anger is scary and destructive, we will physically tighten against anger because our inner truth is that all anger is bad, monstrous, evil, and hurtful. If we believe that any anger is shameful, embarrassing, ugly, and will lead to judgment and rejection, we will panic when we feel it, hold it in, and judge ourselves. We will feel guilty for wanting to right a wrong. We will go through life trying to never be angry. We will forever misunderstand the important messages in anger and even rage.

What we really need is to find the message in the anger. What exactly is it saying? Maybe it's saying, *This is not fair! I deserve to be angry! I need to do something about this!* If we feel too guilty to allow that special brand of *I deserve better* out*rage* for ourselves to rise, we never have the cou*rage* to do something about whatever feels unfair. This is how change happens! We make it happen.

Righting a wrong always involves some degree of anger energy. If we reject anger, we reject our power to make a change. Getting outraged doesn't mean we have to get violent and hostile and punch people in the face or make a scene. It means we allow the energy to come up and flood the third chakra, where it can be used maturely.

Anger gives us the strength, clarity, and willingness to proactively advocate for ourselves. It lifts us into action. That action could be a simple but firm no or setting a clear boundary while asking for exactly what we want instead. It could also mean taking the time to plan out a conversation with someone we have a conflict with and then officially requesting the time to talk it through. Sometimes it means doing the work of following up with necessary facts that support our point of view, getting resources on our side, or starting a movement to solve a bigger problem. Standing up for ourselves when something feels wrong and unfair sometimes just means we make a huge internal decision to use our willpower to change course because the old way is not acceptable.

Generation after generation of people walk around feeling stuck, powerless, and like nothing ever changes. They have no idea the answer to their dilemma is to listen to what their anger is clarifying—what is unfair, what the hurt is, and what it is calling them to do. If we don't have the energy at our third chakra, we're like the hero who gets beaten down again and again by giving in, following the rules, and taking a beating—and then the movie ends.

That's a hard thing to watch, but when we don't have third-chakra energy, all of our words and actions are directed by first-chakra family rules to stay safe. With no anger, there is no courage, and all we have left is freezing or using bonding-response behaviors. We vow to be invisible. We smile, give more, accommodate, cooperate, don't ask for much, and make sure everyone likes us. On the surface these are nice attributes. But inside we feel how these patterns of behavior limit us.

BREAKING THE PATTERN

The first key to breaking this pattern is being aware of how our programming shuts down self-advocacy with self-doubt and guilt. We need to see how we self-block our power in the moment. Self-awareness gives us self-compassion, which sounds like, *Wow, I get it now. I didn't deserve that,* and *I have been programmed my whole life* not *to own my true power.*

The second key is to use the life-changing practice of tapping to safely voice, honor, and move the very intense energies of reactionary anger, rage, hurt, and even hatred. We can't skip this part, and it is important for us to hear how angry we really are and how unfair so much of life has been. This is how we get to know ourselves and what we want in life. This is what gives us permission to have some self-compassion.

Safely leaning into intense emotions with tapping will often release a flood of hurt and tears until a shift happens. This is the big shift of reactionary, messy emotions into the calm strength of what I call leadership energy. A new question can now be felt and answered without regard for the old rules of the comfort zone: *What do I want now?* Whenever we can answer that question, we can call on our leadership energy to make a difference.

LEADERSHIP ENERGY

The goal of our third chakra is to get us to act and inspire change that is in everyone's highest good. When reactionary anger after a hurt is honored and heard, like a child releasing a tantrum, a more mature answer emerges that is always about moving toward something with clarity and certainty. The "bad guy" in our hero story becomes less important, even irrelevant compared to where we are wanting to go next. We set a boundary, say our piece, make our demands, and move on. This is how we know we're in leadership energy.

Leadership energy is leading with authority, authenticity, confidence, and vulnerability all at the same time. We don't question our right to use this energy. It's direct, impactful, and meaningful. We easily admit when we have made a mistake and apologize when necessary because our truth is that we are flawed and human just like everyone else. Setting fair and reasonable boundaries with and for ourselves happens easily and without guilt. Leadership energy is taking bold action with certainty and handling what happens next with courage and honesty.

Leadership energy always carries a win-win intention. Even if that means agreeing to disagree or saying no to someone while saying yes to yourself. The win-win is a calm, conscious, spoken truth that respects the right of all parties to make empowered decisions. The combination of clear boundaries and win-win energy is seen in all great leaders, even in times of difficult conflict or negotiation, and creates unexpectedly positive outcomes. Even when conflicts remain unresolved, we walk away feeling empowered because we honored our integrity.

Third-chakra leadership energy makes us unflappable, as if we have a strong core that makes it hard to knock us off center. With this centered energy, we can handle the critics and the skeptics and enthusiastically speak our truth, on stage and in front of the world if we need to.

When we show up with this energy, it is compelling because it is felt! When we feel it, others feel us! People feel and hear not only what we want or our goal, but they hear the *why*—our passion and realness. They hear the bigger intention in what we want and can get behind it and line up to support us. We inspire passion, enthusiasm, and courage in others because we are allowing them to see and feel the authenticity in us. People respect and respond well to leadership energy. It is true empowerment in action.

Choosing leadership energy over unconscious, reactive energy means not apologizing for being ourselves and instead acting from a place of empowerment. When we release our anger and move with certainty for win-win outcomes, we enroll other people. Those who are aligned with us want to join our mission; those who aren't go their own way. We know that we don't have control over what happens, but we do know that we have every right to take action by showing up and speaking up.

Leadership energy is not something we regret using. At one of my corporate jobs, I went through a hero's journey when someone in management was acting unethically. Most employees knew what was going on, but no one spoke up. I worked with a lot of strong, assertive men, but their first-chakra survival fear ("I can't get fired; I have a family") kept them playing along.

I was a single mom who needed her job, but I eventually found the courage to do something. I knew I could get fired, but I was going to use every bit of my leadership energy to confront the wrongdoing in a prepared, win-win way. In this case my energy was ignited by the compassion I felt for all the co-workers I was speaking up for.

I arranged to meet with upper management and spoke intelligently about the company's ethics policy and mission and about loyalty and care. I stood strong in my certainty and was honest, acknowledging that no situation is ever black-and-white. I addressed the powers that be from a win-win space, and my speech had an impact. I was thanked and changes were made quickly. I used my leadership energy that day, and I have never once regretted it.

COMMENTARY BY DAVID RANIERE, PH.D.

But where we have given of our love and respect not from habit but of our own free will, where we have been disciples and friends out of our inmost hearts, it is a bitter and horrible moment when we suddenly recognize that the current within us wants to pull us away from what is dearest to us. Then every thought that rejects the friend and mentor turns on our own heart like a poisoned barb, then each blow struck in defense flies back into one's own face, the words "disloyalty" and "ingratitude" strike the person who feels he was morally sound like catcalls and stigma, and the frightened heart flees timidly back to the charmed valleys of childhood virtues, unable to believe that this break, too, must be made, this bond also broken.

— Hermann Hesse, *Demian*

At the third chakra we again see the vital role that feelings play in our lives. Here, feelings serve as the fuel needed to compel us into action, and courage is needed to feel them. We tend to talk about courage as something you either have or lack, but I prefer to use action language when describing courage. Courage is something one does or doesn't do in a given moment. It may sound clunky, but I think we *do* courage. And doing the courage to face what feels unfair, and to embrace the anger and hurt unfairness holds, is an incredibly powerful action of empowerment. Without this fuel, action at the third chakra is blocked, thwarted by fear and guilt.

If we think of shame as a painful feeling about who we are, then guilt is how we feel about what we do. So as we move into the action center of the third chakra, guilt is a major player, a powerful countervailing force that opposes empowered action. Like so many other things in life, guilt is complex and neither all good nor all bad. Put simply, guilt is the glue—the bonding compound—that holds relationships together.

Healthy guilt makes us aware of having hurt someone we care about and prompts us to repair ruptures in the relationship. And the stronger the bond, the more painful the guilt. There are few things more agonizing in life than hurting those we love the most.

The psychoanalyst Arnold Modell (1971) has elaborated on two forms of guilt that I find particularly useful in thinking about blockage at the third chakra: separation guilt and survivor guilt. Separation guilt is the deep pain we feel when establishing more distance or a more solid boundary in a relationship. It's a loss of connection, a departure from long-established rules of engagement, or the setting of a different boundary that better serves us and that we have chosen and brought about intentionally (as opposed to other kinds of losses over which we have no control and that do not involve personal agency). It's painful because we are aware that our actions are hurtful to the other person, even if they are right and just.

The Hermann Hesse quote that begins this commentary speaks to this form of guilt and the profound loss and grief that accompany the relinquishment of a deep and long-standing bond. This grief is often a big part of what makes taking action and making changes so difficult; these actions mark a separation from someone we hold close internally, and that separation is felt as a loss. Even if this is a necessary loss in the context of a relationship that is toxic and undermining, the separation will evoke enormous guilt.

We must come to terms with our loss, including the loss of something that has never been but we continue to long for, before we can take the courageous action of either changing or severing the bond. These powerful ties that bind us are often outside of our awareness, and even if we are aware of them, we may not fully appreciate the power of that bond and the price we pay for our loyalty to it.

Survivor guilt is another related form of guilt that can obstruct energy movement at the third chakra. This is the guilt survivors of horrific trauma feel for having survived when others have not. Among the most dramatic examples are combat veterans and holocaust survivors. Much more subtle forms of survivor guilt exist within more normal circumstances, including guilt over "having a better life" than someone we are close to.

Working through these powerful feelings of guilt—and the anger and hurt that it blocks us from accessing—opens up a world of greater freedom. In this world we orient by a future horizon instead of the past and its constraints. The mobilization of empowerment energy at the third chakra forces changes in the prevailing dynamics in a relationship, and paradoxically can often result in a different and more mutually satisfying kind of closeness that is based on authentic engagement rather than guilt.

CHAPTER 10

THE COURAGE TO SAY NO

If the old tribal rules haven't been serving you, it's time to ring out the old rules and ring in a few new ones of your own. Setting boundaries is a necessary skill for living an empowered life. They are a great way to advocate for yourself and honor your true needs, as well as nip draining or toxic relationships or behaviors in the bud. They are clear indicators of how you want and don't want to be treated, and they affirm the certainty of your decisions about what you will and will not do.

In this Healing Experience, you will clear away all your fears of having hard conversations about setting boundaries, and you will practice empowered boundary setting. But because stuck, stewing anger, resentment, and pure fear and guilt (hallmarks of a blocked third chakra) are involved, you may find yourself resisting a bit. That's okay. Just keep at it. This process is the perfect model for dealing with difficult people or preparing for any confrontational situation. You can use it again and again.

Setting a boundary with someone is easy when there is no real problem and you don't expect them to balk at it. This feels more like a conversation about expectations or defining roles. But having to set a boundary with someone because there is a problem is harder. It means something has felt unfair to you, and you expect the other person to push back. This situation requires more energy, certainty, and courage, and those energies only rise up from mature, empowered anger.

I find that many people are not sure what to do or say when they allow their anger to call them to take empowered action. They might feel that burning anger and unfairness, but they aren't sure what to say. Because they have always avoided confrontation, they don't know what will happen next, so they anticipate losing the argument because the other person is too "strong."

"But, Margaret, I don't want to be in a battle. I hate confrontation!" If anger wasn't allowed in your family or if you vowed never to get mad, boundary setting will feel like you have to go into battle. Even thinking about it will make you feel selfish or guilty—just as it did to the hero in the last chapter. You may even worry that you'll be accused of being selfish.

But if you recall, fear and guilt didn't serve our movie hero. They only delayed the time it took for him to get mad enough to put his foot down and set a boundary, so he suffered far more beatings than were necessary. Only by getting angry enough could he get past his guilt, set a boundary, and move into action. However, we are not in a movie where our anger can turn into a badass fight scene. So what can we expect to happen when we stand up for ourselves? By using empowerment energy, we can expect a win-win, or at least to feel whole and right in having said our piece.

In this process, you will build on the rising empowerment energy of the second chakra, especially reactionary anger, and practice how to turn it into leadership energy-in-action at the third chakra. You will also practice it the hard way—with no easy excuses. Just firm, stand-your-ground decisiveness and clarity. You will also see how to move from anger to the win-win energy of a true leader.

HEALING EXPERIENCE #7: THE COURAGE TO SAY NO

Setup Visualization #7-1

Bring to mind someone with whom you need to set a boundary but haven't confronted because you anticipate they'll be difficult to talk to. Think of someone who asks for a lot and is happy taking in a way that, quite honestly, you sometimes resent. You already know that your boundary will make them extremely unhappy, and they will put up a fight. Maybe you have tried to raise the issue before and you ended up fighting, or they poured on the guilt until you ran out of steam and gave in.

Resentment is the hallmark of giving too much and not setting appropriate boundaries. Clients will often say to me, "Margaret, I'm not really mad, I just resent it. After all I do for them, this is how they treat me!" If that resonates as true, then you have chosen the right person for this exercise.

Next take a deep breath, close your eyes, and picture that person on the movie screen of your mind. Notice how they appear to you. Now imagine yourself standing across from them in a future moment when you are about to set a boundary with them.

Let a typical scene with them play out where they are totally doing that thing that they always do, asking or demanding or passively making you do what they want. Only this time you speak up and firmly say no. Furthermore your no has no excuses behind it—no reasons or exceptions to ease the blow. As a matter of fact, you are saying something along the lines of, "No, this does not work for me. I am not doing that. I would rather do my own thing for my own reasons."

Don't worry. I won't really ask you to do this. Just picture it.

Let the scene play out and let the other person react with what would be your biggest fear. How do they look, and what are they saying? What is their energy like? And now notice how you look when they react or overreact to your boundary. Many people first see themselves frozen or blindsided by the other person's reaction, so let's start tapping with that in mind.

Tapping Script #7-1

There they are – And they are not *happy – They are reacting – Just as I feared! – And there I am – Feeling blindsided, attacked – Scrambling, unsure what to say – I can't stand this – I feel angry, I feel scared*

– Unsure what to do – I'm reeling and they are way ahead of me – Getting ready to size me up – And win this one – I can see their face – They're acting shocked – They're acting mad or – They are acting sad and hurt – Maybe they're guilting me or attacking me – Maybe they are trying both at the same time – Talking over me – Drowning me out – Trying to win, trying to put me in my place – Or just get their way – They'll use anger or guilt or both – And if I don't give in soon – It will get worse – Maybe even progress to threats, insults, criticisms – Or maybe they're using their wounding, their Poor me *attitude – And begging me – Demanding just this "one time."*

And I feel it – It feels horrible – A can of worms – I hate confrontation – Now I am in this uncomfortable moment – This is not a win-win moment – It is a win-lose moment – And I am losing – I should have kept my mouth shut – It's going so badly – They always win – And I feel that – Their energy is bigger than mine – Their resolve is bigger than mine – They will debate and fight for hours – And they will not stop until they wear me down – That is why I end up giving in – And they know my weakness – Whether they use anger and escalate – Or use guilt and escalate – They are willing to escalate – To get their way – And I don't matter – They only want what they want.

It is so unfair to me – And they don't want me to change and set a boundary – There they are angry, upset – And coming at me – As if I am crazy – Or as if I am the selfish one – And I am at a loss for the right words – Looking for any exit – I don't like to battle – So I am totally stuck here – This is so unfair – So unfair to me – I feel small and inept – In the face of their force – I can't win – And I am just going to acknowledge how often – This dynamic plays out – And how much it costs me – And drains me – But it takes too much energy to try to change – So I just don't bother.

Post-Tapping Visualization #7-1

Take a breath and notice how true that felt for you. For many it is quite the aha moment to highlight the aspects of the unhealthy pattern with this person out loud.

Tune back into the picture and notice how your mind is painting the scene now. Specifically, does the other person look louder or quieter in their attempts to push back? If they have now gotten more upset and are pushing back harder, tap through that first round again and add in some of the descriptions of how they look and what they are doing to up the ante.

If this person gets explosively angry and this is a very entrenched toxic relationship, recognize first how much this relationship is impacting you, including, if necessary, the naming of the relationship as abusive. Secondly, realize that it may take a lot more work based on the history with this person and their current influence over your life or money.

Keep tapping until you can visualize the image of the two of you in the scene. You want the other person to look calmer, quieter, or less reactive, and you want to feel more solid. The next layer of work is to voice your side of the story regarding how they treat you.

Passive Boundary Setting

With certain people in our life, we might passively set a boundary by letting external circumstances do the heavy lifting. Our misconception is: *In order for me to say no to someone and actually be "selfish," I have to be so overworked, overscheduled, or sick and tired that I can't possibly do what others are asking of me. Only then am I allowed to say, "I'm sorry. I can't do this for you."* It forms a boundary, but it is never from a place of empowerment and means we can't fully choose what we do in life.

Tapping Script #7-2

Now that they look less intimidating – And I feel less manipulated and outgunned – Less intimidated – I can recognize how unfair this is to me – What about what I want? – I am a person too – Not just a resource to be used – I would love to be able to stand up for myself

– And have them hear me – And get it! – I really wanted this to go my way – I need it to go my way – I need to feel as if they heard me – I need to feel that I won – For once – I need them to get it – I need to win – And they need to lose – I want to be victorious – And I need them to see it – To really get it – I want them to hear me – I want them to see the error of their ways – How mean they're being – How uncaring they are acting – How wrong and selfish they are – And I can't say all of that.

But I feel it – That has often been below my words – Even when I smile and go along – Inside I resent it – Inside I would like to win once – And have them wake up – And apologize for everything – And finally change – I need this to work out my *way – I want to them to change – And I want to feel personally validated – That would be so great – I really do want that – I am needing so much – That I can only get from their reaction – So I can finally feel vindicated – I need and want them to validate my experience – And I totally honor that – Part of me would relish winning the argument – And actually enjoy having them lose! – Without that it would never feel fair – So there is actually a lot on the line – That I am not in control of – So I am still feeling anxious, unsure – Afraid of what will happen – I totally honor that.*

Post-Tapping Visualization #7-2

Take a breath and look at the other person again. Check in with how important it feels now that they totally get it, apologize, and accept your truth. How much do you still need that to happen?

Depending on your situation, you may need more rounds of tapping through that script. Sometimes people need to shout and cry their way through the script because it resonates so strongly, whether they are tuning into a teenage child, a pushy friend, or an abusive ex.

This round of tapping voices and honors all the reactionary things you are feeling and wanting out of the process of speaking your truth and setting a boundary. It's an important step because without it you will still be derailed by your frustrations and the unspoken things you wish to "get" from the other person. That keeps you locked in a toxic pattern with them. Without this step you can't hear, honor, and validate your hurts and needs.

When you can validate those for yourself, you go into boundary setting without needing any specific outcome in order to feel that you have spoken your truth. If it now feels less important to get the reaction you would love from them, notice how different you and your energy look in the visualization. Notice how much more solid you feel in your boundary. It is simply your truth.

The best way to go into any difficult conversation or confrontation (it's usually more of a conversation than a confrontation when we tap first) is with the energy that you want to have when it's over. It is human nature to really want someone to validate your experience and apologize, but when it is questionable or unlikely you will get that, you need to take a different tact. It is a powerful process to first honor *for yourself* the unfairness as well as how much you deserve to be treated with respect and care.

When you've let go of anything you need from them in this imagined conversation, that's when you know you're ready to have the conversation from a more empowered, grounded place. When you connect in advance with how you want to feel when it's over—from that empowered, grounded place—your energy will shift and be noticed and felt by you and the other person. A big part of the upside is that they will act differently toward you after this process.

Tune into the scene again and imagine that you are clearly speaking your truth about what you don't like, don't want, or no longer accept, and about what you want and expect instead. Now imagine that this person takes a step toward you and gets louder and more energized, either arguing, cajoling, justifying, or whatever they typically do when you try to set a boundary. In response you simply put your two hands in front of you in the "stop" position and loudly say, "Stop!" You don't have to have the perfect comeback or match their energy or anger. Just see yourself telling this person to stop.

This action is a big piece of your boundary. It is where you energetically disengage from being drawn into the old pattern. Now imagine you say something appropriate for the situation, such as, "This conversation is over if you treat me that way," or "I guess we will have to agree to disagree," or "I can only tell you exactly how I feel and what I want, and right now this is my truth."

Notice how different it is to just stand your ground without reacting by fighting or retreating, which probably always seemed to be your only two options. Yet here you are delivering a calm, centered, unequivocal response without being attached to the outcome. This is leadership energy, and it is your third option. It truly is very much like a wise, patient parent holding a calm boundary with a child who's having a tantrum.

This last round of tapping will allow you to move even more into the third-chakra leadership energy that is less reactive, more self-advocating, and positioned for a win-win whenever possible. You're going to see that your no to them is actually a yes to yourself.

Let's tap again. This time picture them as if you were speaking to them directly.

Tapping Script #7-3

You are over there – And I'm just going to be over here in my energy – With everything that I want to say – That honors me – I honor, I validate – It is my truth – My truth in this moment about this situation – My feelings and the things that I want – I validate them – I honor them – And I release you – I release you – I free you from my need to be right and be validated – I free you to be you – Doing the things the way you do them – And I free myself – To honor my needs – The boundaries I set for myself – And how I want to be treated – All my needs – the things I really want instead – That are a yes to me – I release and free you – Of my need for you to be wrong – Of my need to see you acknowledge – That I'm right and you're wrong – That would be so delicious – And I would love for you to acknowledge that – If this happens, I will accept it graciously – But I honor it for myself – This is my truth – This is what I want – And this is what I do not want anymore – This is my no – That is also a yes to me – I honor this boundary I'm setting with you – And how we interact with and treat each other – So I am setting it as a yes to me – It may change, and I may reset it as needed – But I honor this boundary that is a yes for me.

I free and release you from agreeing with me – You are free to disagree with me – I free you to never see it my way – I would love for you to see it my way – But I free you from my need to enlighten you – That's really hard to let go of – I free you to live the rest of your life – Never understanding me – I honor and free you – And I am open to the highest good – Even though, of course, part of me wants to win – I'm open to a win-win situation – For the highest good for me – And everyone else – Even if it takes time for that to be realized – Even if I never know why it's the highest good for you – I intend the highest good for me first – And for everyone involved, including you – And I free you to say yes to yourself as well – And set your own important boundaries – And make your own empowered choices – I accept all of the consequences that come with this – I honor and bless this whole situation – For the highest good of everyone involved.

Take a breath. How did it feel to say those words? Did you feel the energetic movement into the calm, balanced, and more unattached leadership energy?

Remember to have self-compassion, because you are the hero of your story, and you do deserve better. And as you develop a new habit of being able to manage your feelings and then calmly set and honor boundaries, your whole world will change. Think of the time and energy you will save as your relationships are healed of toxic power plays and simmering unspoken resentments!

Also, it's essential to honor yourself for how incredibly kind, selfless, and giving you are! Yes, maybe to a fault sometimes. But your heart and caring personality should still be honored. Add to that honoring how sacred and deserving you are to be treated with similar kindness, respect, and love.

NEXT STEPS . . .

This week create a list of people in your life you have trouble setting boundaries with and just honor that you have these issues. You don't need to confront anyone. Just be more aware of what you're really feeling because of that and what it's costing you. Then run through this Healing Experience with each person on your list one at a time. It might surprise you how many times just doing this process has led to clients getting honest and sincere apologies from the people they tapped about. Sometimes this process will naturally end up in a conversation or a proactive request for a conversation. If so, tap through all of this again in preparation for that conversation so you can truly be in it with your special brand of win-win leadership energy.

Visit www.unblockedbook.com/chapter10 for an extra tapping experience and discussion to enhance this chapter.

CHAPTER 11

THE COURAGE TO SHINE BRIGHTLY

The National Institute of Mental Health reports that public-speaking anxiety, or glossophobia, affects about 73 percent of the U.S. population. That's hundreds of millions of people. According to the National Social Anxiety Center, the underlying fear is of judgment or negative evaluation by others. Though there is some disagreement on the prevalence, many people experience a racing heart, dry mouth, quaking voice, shortness of breath, and "brain freeze" while speaking in front of a live audience. Public speaking can be a painful inner experience and an embarrassing public one!

I find it complicated to assess how common the fear of public speaking is because so many smart and talented people just avoid it. But why is public speaking so easy for a lucky few who not only seem to enjoy it but make a career out of it? And why do the rest of us either have to work really hard to get over our fear or do whatever we can to avoid it?

We can sometimes chalk the anxiety up to logical factors such as inexperience or lack of preparation. But what about when you are an expert on your topic and you are still terrified? Many of my clients have reported being able to easily present on stage when working for an employer, but when they ventured off on their own and needed to announce their business concept and pricing, they suddenly froze. This was true for me as well and very confusing!

Public speaking requires us to stand up so that our brilliance can be seen and heard. It's akin to enthusiastically shining in the spotlight, boldly owning our gifts, greatness, and authority in our knowledge. And that, dear reader, is why most of us shudder at the thought of getting on stage. Our first- and second-chakra fears trigger the fight-flight-freeze-bond response, and the rest is history.

Some of you will never need to speak on stage, so fear of public speaking may not feel like a burning issue for you. You will still benefit from this Healing Experience because the process will reveal your fears of fully showing up in life.

If you are avoiding public speaking, and your career advancement, salary, or self-employed income depends on it, this fear can and will cost you money. The majority of my clients are following their passions to a new career in which they are the face, talent, and value of their business, and boldly marketing themselves is the difference between thriving or bankruptcy.

In this third-chakra Healing Experience, we're going to use public speaking as an example of how to turn off the fight-or-flight response. To do this we're going to focus not on what people will say if you "put yourself out there" but in the confidence energy you exude. This is the heart of the matter when it comes to anxiety.

We are also going to "heal forward" into the future. Healing Forward uncovers what we truly expect and therefore fear so we can address it directly. With this insight we see fully and clearly exactly how what we learned at the first and second chakras through our hot-stove moments shows up in our adult life. This is how we see the expected tribal punishment that is unconsciously stopping us from taking actions we know we need to take.

Armed with this knowledge, we can shift into that third option again—our third-chakra win-win leadership energy.

HEALING EXPERIENCE #8: THE COURAGE TO SHINE BRIGHTLY

Setup Visualization #8-1

Take a breath and close your eyes, because once again you are going to imagine a scene as if you were in a movie. However, this is a future scene, something that has never happened before but represents putting yourself out there. So imagine yourself in a future moment. You are on a small stage, about to publicly declare your talents and value so you can get a raise or charge more for your services.

Imagine yourself standing there on that small stage surrounded by your family and co-workers, as well as management if you are an employee or a group of potential clients or customers if you are an expert or entrepreneur. For some reason, in this future moment you are filled with confidence and declare loudly and clearly: "I am really, *really* good at what I do! You should listen to what I have to say because I am brilliant and deserve to be paid extremely well for my talents!"

Notice carefully what is happening in this scene. How do the people look? How are they looking at you? How are they reacting, and how do you look and feel?

Some of you will report that your audience looks good, happy, or is even cheering you on. Bravo! This may not be a burning issue for you.

Most of my clients, however, see specific negative reactions from the crowd, even if the audience contains a sprinkle of supportive people. Audience members react to what is underneath the words—the confidence, self-belief, self-value, and boldness. This is critical to reveal because even though you may never say a sentence like that to a group of people, you need to exude that exact energy when you show up, act, and speak. The most common reactions are hostile: your audience will be yelling, laughing, taunting, or accusing you of being selfish or "tooting your horn," all with a *Who do you think you are?* tone. You might see disbelief or skepticism from the crowd or people asking you to "prove it."

This usually triggers fear around whether you are good enough or can prove yourself.

Healing Forward allows us to see our tribal rules manifest—the first-chakra survival fear, where getting rejected by the tribe equals death, and the second-chakra *How dare you!* shaming message. When we allow ourselves to break old rules and show up acting and speaking as though we honor and believe in ourselves, our entire nervous system and thinking mind fully expect the old punishment. This is why we need to jump in and start tapping. As always, feel free to adjust the words to match your inner picture.

Tapping Script #8-1

There I am – Trying to own my power – Bolder than ever – Trying to own my value – Stepping out as me – And this feels like a mistake – It is not safe – They are coming at me – They are not happy – I feel the threat in the air – And it's freezing me – It's very clear – I've made a huge mistake – I want to shrink – I want to hide – Get me out of here.

This is really bad – I wish I had never said that – I feel them pulling away – I have lost them – Or worse, angered them – Irritated them – I can so clearly see – How many don't like my attitude – They are saying, "Who do you think you are?" – They are saying, "Prove it!" – Maybe some are enraged at me – Or laughing, ridiculing me – And I feel it – Who do I think I am? – I don't have the right to act that confidently – Do I?

I am now spinning in self-doubt – I feel humiliated – Embarrassed – Ashamed of acting that way – And my family is there – And they are shocked – Or maybe angry and horrified – I just broke a big rule – And I feel it in my body – They want me to stop – This is not okay for me – There is no way I can handle this – I'm terrified – I'm frozen with terror – It's not safe – It's never been safe – It will probably never be safe – I cannot be confidently me – Shining in the spotlight – That is not allowed for me – No one wants that.

I need to pull this back – I've got to apologize – I'm reeling it all back in – I know how to play whom they need me to be – I feel stuck but safe – It's not safe to be that confident version of me – Not out in the world – I can't say I am special or brilliant – No wonder I play small – No wonder I procrastinate – No wonder I don't ask to be paid more – It's too scary – Too much to risk – Too painful – I can't break those old rules – So I am truly stuck.

Take a deep breath.

Post-Tapping Visualization #8-1

Stuck is the right word, isn't it? Close your eyes and look at the scene again and see what has changed. For some it is worse. Your mind may be painting a picture of a terrifying level of anger, hostility, and personal attack or rejection that, of course, creates panic. If so, keep tapping through that round until you feel calmer and the scene looks calmer and more positive. Keep in mind how much the reaction you expect from the crowd matches the rules and expected punishments you learned at the first chakra level.

When it is calmer and the people seem more receptive, you can move on to another aspect of the third chakra—stubborn refusal. Because the third chakra is our power and action center, it is very strong and willful. But when we feel stuck in a no-win situation and can't lead the way we want to, we will use our third-chakra power to resist and refuse, which looks like procrastination.

Setup Visualization #8-2

There are two sides to procrastination. One side is the *It's not safe* impulse, which we just voiced and honored above. But there's also a long-practiced habit of thinking, *I secretly downright refuse.* Refusing to be seen as powerfully you is a *huge* energetic withholding of you, your light, and your gifts. Think about it: Is that good in any part of life?

Let's tap through the points on this.

Tapping Script #8-2

This is exactly what I was afraid of – This is why I hold back – And obviously I am right – Even though I probably could speak – Why should I? – They're just going to judge me – Pick me apart – They're a bunch of skeptics – Maybe it seems some are willing to listen now – But I don't trust them – I know how judgmental people are – They're going to size me up – And try to trip me up – And I'll feel like a fool – And the truth is – I can't back up these claims of brilliance – Brilliance is not my birthright – It is something proven and earned – And I don't know for sure whether I am good enough yet.

I have not earned that confidence yet – They could call me on this – And I will be standing there – With my mouth hanging open – Stuck and frozen – Like a fraud – They will judge me – Criticize me – Pick me apart – Now I'm not talking – I refuse to talk – I refuse to "shine" – I'm going to stay silent – And keep this on my list but refuse – It is safer for me – I am safer from judgment – If I just withhold myself – Let someone else take the spotlight – Let someone else put themself on the line – Let someone else earn the big money – I'm going to hold back – That's the smarter thing to do – It's not safe – And I know myself – I cannot handle criticism – I'll be humiliated and embarrassed – I will crumble – It has happened before – Then I will beat myself up forever – I can't handle it – I'm not going to talk – I am going to stay silent – I can be stubborn about this – You want to see third-chakra willpower? – I've got it.

Take a deep breath. How did it feel to voice that side of your strength?

Many people say, "You know, I have a fear of standing out. I have a fear of being successful. I am afraid of owning my power." And there is truth in that, but underneath it is an absolute, stubborn refusal to own that power. Combined with the real wounds at the first chakra that create the real fears, the real hurts, the real rejections that happened at some point a long time ago, there is a practiced habit of holding back. Something is needed to break through that third-chakra block, and it is always passion!

How badly do you really want to change and why? Are you passionate about your goals? Do you care about stepping up into the next chapter of your life, with you shining with confidence, giving your gifts, making a real difference, and being paid well for that? Are you sick of being stuck, playing small, and watching your life go by? Are you angry and irritated enough about what the old way is costing you that you want to push harder? Feel into that and let it rise. *That* is passion. The *I want this, and I deserve to have it* fuel from the second chakra rising up to fill the third chakra with the energy to lead your life forward.

Let's voice some of that and see how it impacts your energy!

Tapping Script #8-3

The truth is – I am sick and tired of being stuck – I hate it – I can't move forward – And I want to – There are so many things I want – So many things I want to do and receive – Why can't it finally be time for me? – Why can't this be my time? – Time for me to rise – And own my power – To be fierce and courageous – I am sick of giving away my power – I hate when I do that – I am sick of being underpaid and undervalued – F__ that! – Enough already – I am sick of hiding – While others take the spotlight – Yes, I have fears and self-doubts – Because I am human – But I want to claim my right to shine – I want to claim my right to be heard and seen – I want to claim my right to own my brilliance, gifts, and experience – I have it all – But I am so stuck in the old ways – And that is devastating – I am so angry about it – Really angry about it – And resentful too – I have given so much – Accommodated so much – Always been a team player – Taken advantage of – And underappreciated – And I hate that – No more – No more – No more – I am putting my foot down with myself – For real – I will not be contained anymore – No more unconscious fears – No more ridiculous rules from the past – I am not a child anymore – I have so much potential – So much to do and be – And I am done wasting time.

Feel the energy in your body after voicing that. Notice how it is a filling, charging-up battle-cry energy designed to move and motivate! This is empowerment energy moving up into the third chakra, setting a boundary with your internal rules and calling you to lead with action. Feel that, move with it, and notice the kinds of actions you feel compelled to take right now.

Setup Visualization #8-4

This last round of tapping will introduce a mature, balanced leadership energy of power and vulnerability. You can tap through this round and use it again and again by simply closing your eyes and imaging yourself saying it to any group you need to speak in front of.

Take a breath, close your eyes, and come back to the picture of you on stage again. This time let your family or others fade from the picture and leave only the people who represent perfect potential customers, clients, or bosses.

Tapping Script #8-4

The truth is – I am awesome at what I do – I am brilliant and expert – And I am also not perfect – Of course I am not perfect – I am human – I am really passionate about my mission and goals – I am valuable and totally deserve to be paid well – And yet not perfect – I don't know everything – I am still learning new things like everyone else – But I know my stuff – Even though I can still make mistakes and will never be perfect – I know my stuff – And I have all this experience – And I really, really *care – I love fixing problems – I love bringing solutions – I am passionate about what I do – I actually love it – Even though I get nervous sometimes – And totally doubt myself.*

Oh well; I am human – But from the bottom of my heart, I invite you – Because I am an expert and I do care – And I can help you – Some of you – Who have the specific problems I know how to solve – And I give you permission to not be interested – If this does not apply to you – I give you permission to not resonate with me at all – That is okay – I may not be the right fit – I am here to help those who are needing help – And are the right fit – And I give all *of you permission – To be both awesome* and *human too – I give all of you permission to shine with your gifts – And to not have to be perfect – I give all of you permission to totally own your value – And believe in yourselves enthusiastically – Even if you still have human fears, self-doubts, and imperfections – Just like me – I am here for win-win awesomeness – And I intend the highest good for all.*

Take a breath and notice how different that felt. This is the third option—your leadership energy. When we can enthusiastically shine as who we are, both awesome and flawed, we give everyone permission to do the same. That's why it feels so good to be around people who are enthusiastically being themselves. Again, though we would likely never say those exact words, it is the beautiful energy and intention we can consciously carry underneath everything we do and say, especially when we market ourselves. Imagine if you were to show up with that energy!

NEXT STEPS . . .

This week I'd like you to reconnect with your passion for your next new chapter. For example, why did you buy this book? What do you really want to do, be, and give? Next, start practicing ways that you can show up and shine. Think of one thing you can do to step out and be seen in a bigger way around your passion or goals, even if it's a baby step. Then pick some supportive friends who love you and practice being more enthusiastically you with them. Not the perfect you but the real, amazing, imperfect, silly, smart, flawed, sweet you—all of you!

Visit www.unblockedbook.com/chapter11 for an extra tapping experience and discussion to enhance this chapter.

CHAPTER 12

THE COURAGE TO BE YOUR AUTHENTIC SELF

"I was feeling so good about myself! I had really stepped up and started telling my family about how exciting it was . . . until my sister said, 'Well, aren't you full of yourself?'"

Talk about deflation! I have heard hundreds of versions of this story. It's as if certain people know our weak spots and just go for blood, and we feel it. The slap-down of the old rules rises again!

By now you have built up a new level of empowerment energy that can carry you into new places both within yourself and out in the world. But stepping up and being seen more as your authentic self—or the person you are growing into—is new and must be practiced. You will experience setbacks—and pushback, like in the anecdote above—as you flex this new muscle. Your current tribe may not be in a place to totally understand and support you as you own your power. When we lose our power at the third chakra, we lose our will and courage, and that can lead to procrastinating on taking small but important steps toward our goals and dreams.

In this chapter we're going to work on third-chakra resiliency so you can handle setbacks, pushback, and even haters who don't exactly cheer for your new level of confidence. We will again use the approach I call Healing Forward to uncover and pre-empt future potential blows to your budding inner confidence. You can practice how to more solidly stand your ground with grace, respect, and leadership, even in the face of criticism.

We will also use this work to show you how to get unstuck, out of procrastination, and into effective, focused, bold action. You'll end this session with a more powerful and grounded inner sense and voice about your value, gifts, and courage.

HEALING EXPERIENCE #9: THE COURAGE TO BE YOUR AUTHENTIC SELF

Setup Visualization #9-1

We are going to build directly on the previous Healing Experience but add in some new elements. First I want you to bring to mind something you have been avoiding doing that you know you need to do. It should be something that is an important step toward your goals and that would have a big impact. Procrastination can take many forms—you could be feeling brain fog about what to do next, zoning out, or keeping yourself busy or distracted doing other things. Sometimes we can convince ourselves or others that we're not procrastinating, so really check in on this.

Now imagine I show up at your home and announce that I am going to stand there while you do this task, and you have to do it right now—today! Notice whatever resistance is coming up in you. It could feel like anxiety, stress, or even anger.

Let's start tapping and once again voicing that third-chakra stubborn refusal.

Tapping Script #9-1

Ugh! – I really don't want to do this – I don't want to do it – This is stressing me out – And I am feeling it – And now there is pressure – And I am being forced to do it – And I am feeling it – I have so much resistance to doing this – That is why I have been avoiding it – And though that is driving me crazy – I can now feel how much I dread it – I don't want to do it – It does not feel safe somehow – Though I think it should be easy – And other people seem to do it easily – I feel dread – It does not feel safe – I don't like this – I don't want to do it – And what if I fail? – What if I publicly fail? What if my efforts don't work? – Or people don't like it? – There are so many things I am worried about – What if it goes badly? – I totally honor that underneath my procrastination – Something about this feels scary – Even though the task should be doable – There is actually a lot at stake for me.

Post-Tapping Visualization #9-1

Take a breath and notice how you feel. What is at stake for you? What are you worrying about? Regardless of what it is you have to do, there is always a fear that has at its core how exposed you will be to other people's judgments and criticisms—and your own. What is the worst-case scenario?

Now take a breath and get ready to close your eyes because we are about to imagine the scenario where that very bad thing happens. Imagine now that you could see yourself in a future moment when you have been successfully forced to take that action. It should be easier to see that happening after that refusal tapping round. Allow your mind to paint the picture of how that action is being seen and experienced by other people in a way that makes sense in your situation.

If you are making a video, for instance, you can picture people out in the world watching your video. If you are making a sales call, picture the person answering you on speakerphone. See yourself doing your best; being honest, sincere, and caring; and possessing all the positive vibes from the last chapter. Let yourself be in that *I am awesome* vibe. Just be with that for a minute.

But now the scene changes as a person publicly declares, "You are not special! You are nothing! I *know* you!" Then this person calls you out on your biggest fear and source of secret self-doubt. Note exactly what they say. Check in with your body and notice where you feel what just happened.

Let's start tapping.

Tapping Script #9-2

Wow – *That really hurt; I really felt that – I feel it in my body – Especially in my* __________ *– This is really hard – This does not feel good – Felt like an attack – Angry, hostile – And it* was *an attack – A public takedown – My worst nightmare – And I felt it – Right in my core – And I feel deflated and so hurt – It's so shocking – So horrifying – And so mean – And now I am reeling – Shamed publicly – Clearly, I just failed big time.*

I am angry, and I could cry – I mean, screw you! *– And now I wish I never spoke this – This is why I avoid doing certain things – Here it is: my worst nightmare – And I'm feeling it – The fear – The shame – The sadness – This has already been stopping me – And it may actually happen someday – And this is how bad it will feel – And I feel how it hits me in my core – Of course I have to feel those words! – And I feel them – And they trigger my deepest self-doubts – I worry inside already that I am not good enough – I mean, what if I am nothing? – Not important – And not good enough – This is intolerable – Ugh!*

I've carried this for a long time – And it's been costing me for a long time – This fear of standing in my power – Because I might have to face – Something so terrifying – So shaming – Something I am secretly so afraid of – What if I am nothing? – What if I am not *special? – I'm going to honor all of this right now – I honor all of my feelings – And the programming in my nervous system – And the fear I learned as a child – To never break this rule – About standing out and acting as if I am special – As if I deserve – Acting as if I have the right to be heard and seen – I'm just going to see it and honor it.*

Take a deep breath. We have built up to this point chakra by chakra, working to heal and understand the foundation of your unconscious actions and how you limit your power. We have arrived at real-life adult situations that can and do play out, both in our minds and in life as we start to step out of our comfort zones.

It has always been my commitment to prepare my clients for their secret worst-case scenario in advance in a safe, supportive way. It's hard and intense, but this is what builds the new muscle of trusting yourself to handle and recover from big setbacks. Self-trust is the cornerstone of third-chakra resilience.

Post Tapping Visualization #9-2

Take another breath and tune into your big goal or mission and how this one micro-task that you have been avoiding is important in making that goal happen. Now I want you to do something very strange: Give yourself permission right now to never take that step at all. Give yourself permission to completely let go of your dreams, goal, mission, and all the pressure you have put on yourself to charge forward, change, and get things done. I call this going down the "no road." Breathe into that and notice how that feels.

The truth is you don't *have* to do anything. Most people, even when extremely passionate about their goals, feel a huge sense of relief and lightness when they have this permission. You can even say out loud, "I don't *have* to do anything!"

This little exercise takes people by surprise, but this what it is like to be an empowered adult. You make conscious decisions about what you want and don't want, and you live fully conscious of the consequences of your decisions.

So imagine yourself letting go of your dream, and watch how that looks and feels over the next five years. Take in the good and the bad and however that feels for you. Don't rush it. Be with everything it means and entails.

After a few minutes, come back to the present moment and then go down the *Yes, I want this* road and see all the things that may play out—the good and the bad and the peaks and the valleys. But because this yes road means you are stepping way out of your old rules, fears, and comfort zones, you have to include possibilities of what might happen. Most important, you need to imagine people you have not met yet who will likely be a big part of your new journey and will arrive because of the empowered energy you are carrying and the authentically-awesome-while-still-being-human *you* that you are being. Given that, you must be open to the possibility that these yet-unknown people will likely become extremely important to you and to your mission and goals.

Now decide which road you want and which road you don't want. This is not a lifelong, constraining decision. Things can change. This is simply your right-now, in-this-moment, gut-check decision. Can you reaffirm inside that you really do want your goal, even with how hard this part of the work is, or is it time to let your goals and dreams go?

Let's tap again.

Tapping Script #9-3

I really do want this – But it's scary to want it – It's scary to voice it – I'm not sure I can really ask for it – Not with my full voice – I don't want to get my heart broken – I don't want to be disappointed – Of course I don't! – I don't want to be judged – Or attacked – No one does! – So I am just going to honor – That I'm kind of afraid to want it – It's scary to really want it – It's scary to express that – To say that I want it more than to survive – To say that I want to have this big energy – And maybe even impact more people with my gifts – To let myself really want that – I learned a long time ago – That it's dangerous to really want – To really want my deepest needs.

And I am really seeing how that plays out – In my adult life – How I unconsciously avoid breaking old rules – And instead only want things that are more appropriate – Only act and speak in ways that people wouldn't judge me for – That I have learned are safe – That didn't ruffle any feathers – I totally get it now – How much I strive – To protect myself from criticism – And from disappointment – I didn't want to get my heart broken – Of course I don't – No wonder I am procrastinating on this small step – Because there is so much at stake for me.

But the truth is – I really do want this – This is my mission – This is my goal – And I've danced around it – But the truth is – I really do want this – For a lot of reasons – And I have so much I want to do and give – And so much of an impact to make – And I want it because it will be awesome – It will be fun – It will be freedom – That I've wanted for so long – And in exchange, yes, I am willing to show up – And give my best – Strive to be my best – I love giving my gift – And I want to give it to more people – I want to give my gift in a bigger way – That allows me to receive in bigger ways too – Maybe even earn more money – Be seen and validated for my efforts and courage – Bigger.

The truth is – I have all sorts of fears and insecurities – Of course I'm afraid of failure – But too bad; I'm going for it – I'm letting myself want it – And I'm going for it – I've been stuck for so long – I'm done playing small – It's still scary, but I'm done playing small – This is my time now – This is my mission – This is my gift, and I want to give it – I'm still afraid – I'm totally insecure at times – Sometimes I'm lazy – Sometimes I make dumb mistakes – And I'm going to worry about judgment – Of course I am – I'm totally human – But I have also been incredibly brave in my life – Brave and courageous – And I have been extremely strong – And I can be super stubborn when I need to be – I have overcome a lot of hard stuff already – So I do believe in myself – And I do want it – And despite the ups and downs I know will come – I'm still going for it – This is my mountain, and I'm going to climb it – This is my time.

Take a deep breath.

How does it feel? How did those words feel? More important, how does it feel in your body now, and what do you feel ready to do and be?

Post-Tapping Visualization #9-3

Take a minute to revisualize yourself taking action on that task and see what is different. How do you look in the picture, and how do the people observing you look? Now imagine that person stands up to speak their venom. How do you handle it, and how do the rest of the people look at that person?

It's important to take note of what images your mind is showing you regarding the shift that has taken place internally. Imagine that person can be welcomed to leave, since they have no positive reason to stay. Notice again how you look.

A common, immediate response is to see yourself looking more "solid." That is what we are looking for. Even when others push back and it's unexpected and hurtful, we can still be solid in who we are—in our gifts, mission, and intention.

Imagine taking action now with that kind of energy, centeredness, and certainty!

NEXT STEPS . . .

This week practice what it is like to self-reveal with safe, supportive people in your life. It is one thing to tap on this alone in your home to heal and move the energy, but it needs to be practiced with a real person.

Start by choosing someone who already loves you, believes in you, and supports your empowerment. This should be someone capable of holding this space for your greatness and humanity. Ask them to do a little face-to-face exercise with you. Not by phone but in person or by video chat.

Begin by reading something you have prepared that explains the specifics of your goals and dreams, why you are passionate about them, and all the gifts you bring to those goals and dreams. This is hard, but you must read an extensive list of your qualities and experience. And breathe, because this will be challenging.

Then you must tell them about your no-road and yes-road visualizations, including what you saw and how they helped you become more decisive. Finally, using the tapping script above, tell them about all the ways you are flawed and at the same time uniquely qualified and ready for your mission. For example, you might explain how you are scared at times and even weak *and* how you can be incredibly strong and brave.

When you are done, allow the other person to share whatever they want to share with you without interruption. While they talk you must work to stay present and *let it in*, which will be the hardest part of all. To help you stay present, keep breathing, tap on your collarbone spot, or place your hand over your heart while you listen, if you'd like.

When they are done, ask them: If the worst thing happened and you put yourself out there and it went really badly or someone attacked you with harsh words, how would they support you? What would they do or say to you if something like that happened?

As part of our new strength and resiliency, we need to break the habit of isolating and going quiet when bad things happen. Instead we need a safe space to reach out for loving support from our consciously chosen adult tribe of real friends who have our back. Now on solid ground, we feel safe to launch out into the world anew.

As you finish, thank them for being there for you.

Visit www.unblockedbook.com/chapter12 for an extra tapping experience and discussion to enhance this chapter.

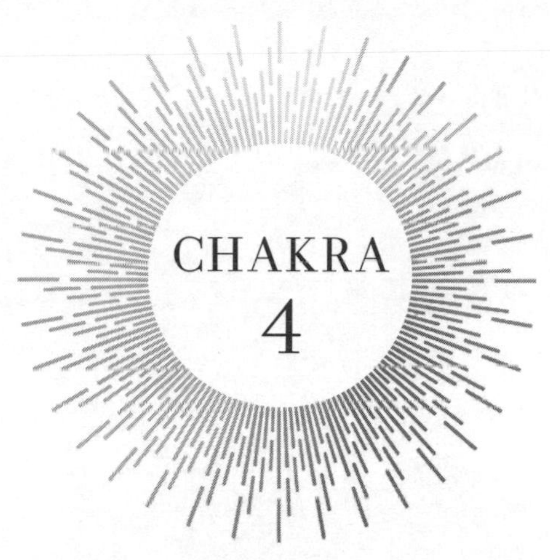

THE POWER OF SELF-LOVE—HEALING THE HEART CHAKRA

Imagine . . . that your automatic reaction
to taking *bold*, imperfect action
always sounded like . . .
"Look at how great *I did*!
(And I look *fab* too.)" Yes, seriously.

CHAPTER 13

RADICAL RECLAIMING OF SELF-LOVE AND ACCEPTANCE

Imagine you're browsing through some shelves at your parents' house, and you come across a dusty old tape with a handwritten label. It's a video of you at the age of four in a dance recital. You haven't seen the tape in ages. Curious, you blow off the dust and push the video in the slot of your parents' ancient VCR, sit down on the couch, and give it your full attention.

You're so cute! You and the other kids are out of sync and repeatedly making eye contact with your instructor, a sure sign that you have no idea what to do next. You stumble, maybe even fall, as you transition from one move to the next, but you are clearly enjoying yourself, oblivious to your missteps. You smile as you watch your joyful enthusiasm, only seeing yourself as precious and lovable, even as you make all kinds of mistakes in front of your audience. You lovingly chuckle and feel the joy of who you were at that moment—with total acceptance of your flaws and all.

How many of us can say we look at our present-day selves the same way? Most of us don't feel joy or laugh at our mistakes or subpar performance. We beat ourselves up in very practical-, rational-, and logical-sounding ways, telling ourselves we should have known better, done it better, or been smarter or more perfect. Add to that the times when we "should" have been stronger, such as when we gave in to someone's pressure to do something we didn't want to do or laughed along when someone insulted or made fun of us.

In these situations we tend to be much less forgiving of ourselves. We have no compassion for any suffering or hurt we endured and certainly no forgiveness for what we see as our part in past situations—just harsh criticism that starts as soon as we get through the moment. We chastise ourselves for being weak—again. *Why didn't I stand up for myself?* we ask repeatedly inside our heads. We take the anger that is naturally triggered at the situation and turn it against ourselves as shame. And if we do eventually blow up at other people, we end up feeling embarrassed and humiliated for acting foolishly. Either way it is a no-win situation because we blame ourselves. Forgiving ourselves comes less easily. We'll likely replay the scenario in our heads for years, as if it were a tape recording that won't quit.

Amazingly, we don't realize that we are playing a recording. We do it automatically and never question why we do it or what the negative consequences might be to our energy, confidence, or self-worth. This self-criticism and lack of self-compassion are habits we've completely normalized inside our heads. If someone pointed it out to us, or suggested being easier on ourselves, we would roll our eyes at how naive or wrong they are. We might smile and nod politely. We know, however, that we are "right" to criticize ourselves, because our standards for ourselves are high, even if we would never be that hard on someone else. We would argue that we deserve and need that criticism because it's the truth—our truth.

This is the powerful, amazing, all-encompassing Heart Chakra in action—the good, the bad, and the ugly. It's where we find the glorious faculties of love, compassion, and forgiveness, the light side of the heart that allows us to connect with and adore our four-year-old self despite our mistakes. It's where we're capable of beholding ourselves, or entering into a sacred relationship with ourselves that doesn't want to fix, change, or judge but simply witness the divine energy within. The Heart Chakra knows we deserve all good things. But it's also got a dark side none of us can underestimate.

Because the heart has so much power, a critical Heart Chakra can be the darkest, meanest, cruelest, and worst place of all. This is the heart's closed and false dark side. The dark side lives and breathes on deep-seated and unacknowledged grief caused by big and small traumas. This part of the Heart Chakra is self-scrutinizing. It won't let us forgive ourselves or others for past mistakes or pains. Our dark side reminds us daily, hourly, and even by the minute about the many circumstances in which we should have been better, smarter, and stronger but weren't. When the heart operates by this critical, dispassionate energy, we're guided not by the heart's compassion but by the heart's biggest, most destructive, and least questioned force: false wisdom.

Characteristics of the Heart Chakra

The Heart Chakra is the fourth level of consciousness in the chakra system. It is the home of wisdom, joy, love, and compassion for the self and others, and *true* acceptance of every aspect of ourselves—every impulse, every mistake, every less-than-perfect part of us. Located smack-dab in the middle of the seven chakras, the Heart Chakra is positioned to deliver lower-chakra energy straight through to the top chakra, or Crown Chakra. When our energy moves full-on with heartfelt compassion, we have the most to offer—and to gain. Whatever we create, say, or do (or don't do) is for the highest good. An open heart, when fueled by the lower three chakras, can move mountains in our lives and in the lives of those we touch. Here's where we can truly feel empowered.

The Heart Chakra is what I call the wise integrator of the true self. It is capable of bringing all the chakras together to make us feel whole. When we fully tune in to our heart, all other systems become synced. When our chakras are integrated, we accept each chakra, dark sides and all, as sacred. Balance is central to the Heart Chakra: masculine/

feminine, dark/light, yin/yang. That's why we sometimes see polar-opposite behaviors in ourselves. One minute we're the warrior woman, and the next we're the damsel in distress. This dynamic range of the Heart Chakra gives our nature the space it needs to unfold.

FALSE WISDOM: THE TRUTH BE TOLD

False wisdom is an inner-belief system driven by half-truths, lies, and misguided ideas about what it means to be a good and worthy person. It feels like self-righteousness—that sense of being right—because, well, logically, we *are* right. We *were* completely unprepared for that dance recital, we *shouldn't* have laughed nervously when we were insulted, and we *shouldn't* have caved into another's wishes, and there are a million ways we *could* have done it differently or better. False wisdom is not wise at all, but it sure sounds smart. It's got some compelling facts and stories to back it up, after all.

False wisdom is supported by the belief that improving our faulty selves is more important than anything else, including forgiveness and compassion. Forgiveness and compassion are only for some future moment when we have finally learned our lesson and are doing everything right.

Improving, on the other hand, means we need our mistakes and faults to be constantly reviewed and pointed to as a warning so we never forget. This serves as a form of insurance so we never stop stressing and worrying about doing things right because that would lead to slacking off. False wisdom's conclusion is that we need to be continually driven by anxiety, self-doubt, and reminders that we are somehow broken until we are fixed and improved enough to finally measure up to a preprogrammed standard of perfection. Only through that achievement of perfection will we finally get to feel lovable, joyful . . . or good enough. Only through that ultimate achievement will we finally deserve to rest and allow in love from others, celebration, and the receiving of all good things.

False wisdom, then, is when *our inner critic becomes our inner coach*. Whew! Think about that for a moment. It's the fuel of the heart's dark side, which insists that we're seeing the whole picture, even though that is far from the truth. It's as if you looked at that dance recital tape, pulled it out in anger, and slammed it on the floor, refusing to watch something so stupid and unprofessional. Never mind that you're only four! It's not terribly different from the aftermath of rape or other sexual abuse, when victims don't see the bigger picture or all the factors involved. They only see the million ways *they* should have done something different. They are full of self-blame, focusing on why they didn't stand up for themselves or why they didn't fight harder. That sounds so cruel, but we don't see it as the dispassionate cruelty to ourselves that it is.

False wisdom packs a powerful punch. It beats us up every day. When we hold fast to the false wisdom of the inner critic, we close up and block our beautiful heart energy and instead live in our heads, evaluating ourselves and others rather than feeling some of life's greatest joys.

Hidden behind false wisdom is something most would never expect: grief. Hidden behind the "just the facts" practicality of our self-judgments are pockets of hidden, unacknowledged grief that hold our anger, shock, hurt, and a whole bunch of loss.

The Cost of a Weak Fourth Chakra

- Struggling to feel yourself at your core
- Feeling as if something has been missing in your life for a long time
- Giving of yourself freely but can't receive
- Feeling empty inside instead of joyful, even when achieving big things
- Feeling secretly lonely and on your own, even within a relationship
- Holding back your true feelings

- Reacting unconsciously
- Acting overly responsible for everything and everyone
- Criticizing yourself for each and every thing that you could have done better, even when others celebrate you
- Seeming incapable of letting in praise and compliments
- Having trouble accepting true support but opting to be stronger and soldier on
- Doing everything yourself or micromanaging (i.e., seeing others as helpless children)
- Holding your anger inside and instead dismissing people with your unspoken judgments
- Having a secretly tender but guarded heart
- Not being "felt" by others—people don't feel your passion or how much you care
- Lacking connection with others because they can't connect with or feel your intention to help them

Benefits of a Strong Fourth Chakra

- Experiencing the self, everything, and everyone as they truly are—beautiful, perfect, and infinitely lovable and deserving of all good things
- Feeling the magnificent warmth and "field presence" of the undefended heart that has the capacity to love
- Living in the expanded, amazing freedom of true self-acceptance (and freedom from the relentless inner critic)

- Seeing the pure divinity of yourself and others
- Being a healing force by just being yourself, as people shift from their dark to the light just by being in your presence
- Allowing your compassion, softness, caring, and heartfelt intentions to be heard and felt by others

GRIEF: THE UNCRIED TEARS OF THE HEART CHAKRA

In *Eastern Body, Western Mind,* author Anodea Judith teaches that the "demon" of the Heart Chakra is grief. I have found that most people only relate to the grief of losing people in their life or of having a broken heart from a romantic relationship. Grief from the loss of another is commonly understood and socially acceptable, and we give people space and compassion to heal, often through traditional rituals or expected behaviors. For example, if your best friend just lost her husband, you would expect her to go through a grieving process—to be in shock, cry, feel sad, and be angry. You would understand if, at a major holiday two years after this death, your friend got teary-eyed. You wouldn't tell her to "get over it already."

But there is another type of grief we carry that is not recognized or given space for—those pushed-down pockets of grief that have never been heard, held, and healed. This is the grief that is at the root of false wisdom. This variety of grief is buried deep below our mind's rational thinking, and we do not know it is there. It is the grief of uncried tears. And it is *always* hidden underneath ruthless self-judgment and criticism, or false wisdom, making it seem like a victimless crime.

To get a clearer picture of the consequences of unacknowledged grief, imagine a boy going up to bat in a Little League game. He loves the sport and enjoys being outdoors with his friends and having fun, until he strikes out three games in a row. From then on, when the boy goes up to bat, his coach is standing next to him, criticizing and belittling him: "Gonna do it right this time? You didn't do it last week. You're the reason we always lose. Are you going to have another bad game?" Then the boy gets a cell phone, and his coach texts him twenty-four hours a day. From the moment he wakes up until he goes to bed at night, the boy reads his coach's messages: "Awful day yesterday. Gonna do better today or mess up like yesterday? You should have done it better."

That's incredibly harsh, ruthless, and mean, right? Imagine how that boy's excitement about playing is going to disappear and be replaced by stress, anxiety, and bracing for criticism. Eventually we would expect that child to break down into tears as the criticism wears him down. Well, that coach is no different from our inner critic. That's what it does to us 24/7/365. We have just stopped feeling the pain and the tears that would flow, and instead believe it is the truth. It beats the joy and fun out of us and out of life, leaving us to believe that we are not good enough. And every time it does that, we hurt deeply. It breaks our hearts, but we are so locked in on the habit, we don't feel the heart pain it is causing.

Superachievers are notorious for having a huge well of uncried tears, but they have no idea they're carrying around so much grief. Their inner critic is part of what drives them to be so accomplished, and they kind of admire it. Their inner critic sounds logical, full of evidence, and right: *Yes, I should have done better.* But these messages are not victimless crimes. They are ruthless, mean energy directed at the self. They embody a refusal to be self-compassionate, patient, and understanding. They demand to reach impossible standards and won't acknowledge that they're doing their best, much less celebrate any progress. Underneath that is the hurt of hearing that *you* don't have value; it's only what you do that matters.

If I bring up the subject of buried grief to clients, they adamantly deny having any. They will deny it until they are blue in the face. They aren't lying; they just don't know it's there. They've managed to muscle over the pain to keep it buried. They want to be more in their power, but they can't feel their heart, their life, or their core. This is the true cost of frozen grief hidden under a constant inner critic. They always feel as if something's missing—and that something is *them.*

The Big R: Resistance

When and if we start to become aware of this type of grief, our practical, rational mind will raise huge resistance. We will feel an urgency to push it down. Of all the emotions, buried grief is the one we are least willing to feel.

To block the voice of that grief, here is what our rational mind will say:

What is the point of feeling this? It's not going to change anything. The past is the past. (This thought will come with resignation.)

If I let myself feel this, it will be too big and overwhelm me. I may never stop crying, or worse, I may become depressed and unable to do anything. So it's not safe to grieve. (This thought will come with a strong sense of fear.)

If I start feeling all this grief, I will be ineffective and inefficient. I don't have time for all that weakness. (This thought will come with determination and righteousness.)

Does any of this sound familiar?

WHERE'S THE GRIEF?

When we can finally find, voice, honor, and move that grief, watch out! The inner critic loses its space in our head—and it packs up all its false wisdom with it. To heal the Heart Chakra, we must find where we have pushed down pockets of hurt and grief. Tapping is the most effective way I know to get past our defensive structures of trying not feel painful emotions and to voice, honor, and move buried grief.

Where do we find this grief? In two distinct places.

The first place is where our deepest wounds lie—heartbreaking betrayals by others, particularly those whom we trusted, including parents, spouses, and other loved ones. Usually these are the stories we are aware of and may have even told many times in our lives to friends or therapists—stories we lived through and have lived with. We see these wounds as our history that we must accept and are often totally disconnected to the real impact they have had on us.

Wounds from our parents are always inflicted in the context of what was normal and normalized in our childhood, and that makes them hard to see. Whether we see these wounds as unforgivable—and we've no intention of letting the offender off the hook—or we make excuses for our wounders out of loyalty, we don't usually see what good could come from revisiting them. We learn to live with them, with no way to voice our anger and hurt and have it be heard, validated, and held with love. Without this true healing, they continue to cost us day in and day out, creating anxiety, self-doubt, perfectionism, fear of intimacy, fear of betrayal, low self-worth, and more.

The second place where we find unacknowledged grief is hidden beneath our smart-sounding inner critic. We must work directly with, not against, our inner critic to get past the distorted mirror of flaws it is fixated on. This is when we break through, touch the compassion in our heart, and can truly heal. So we must go to the secret places where we are hard, unaccepting, not compassionate, rejecting, and totally impatient with *ourselves*. I call them secret because they truly are blind spots. We don't see them as areas of pain and grief but as something that we are right about. This justifies our self-criticism, the recording we play over and over in our heads.

Voicing, honoring, and moving grief and crying our uncried tears refills the Heart Chakra from the inside out with pure love. The more grief we release, the more love we get!

THE HEART AS HEALER

So far this book has taken you through nine processes of healing at the first three chakras. My guess is that you've experienced a greater flow of energy in your body and your life. You're seeing results. So you may be surprised to learn that all the healing you've experienced has happened in the light side of the Heart Chakra. It's worked, even if your Heart Chakra energy is at an all-time low, because my scripts have been modeling how I want you to treat yourself. Like a kind and caring parent, I've been holding Heart Chakra energy for you by gently guiding you through each process and creating a safe space for you to heal.

Even when a script has asked you to think or view harsh words or images, you have felt safe. I wasn't judging you. I waited patiently until you were done. I didn't tell you to hurry up and get over it already. By asking you to call up imagery from your unconscious mind, I wasn't putting you or anyone else in a dangerous situation. You knew no one was going to get hurt and that no blood would be spilled. I wasn't having you confront your arch-enemies face-to-face in real life or making things worse by creating more grief, pain, and resentment.

The light side of the Heart Chakra is so beautiful because it doesn't judge or criticize even the harshest of the words you've been reciting in these scripts. It acts as a witness—during breakdowns, temper tantrums, bursts of anger, you name it. It allows you to finally get into the grief. It lets you heal and watches as the divine energy within you unfolds. Everything we've done so far has been supported by love and compassion—by the best of the Heart Chakra. And it's had a qualitative depth to it. Telling you to think positive thoughts while you carry a surge of negative feelings doesn't address the root of the problem—the grief. It's putting frosting on a moldy brownie.

In some people whom we might consider to be spiritually advanced, for instance, the light and dark sides of their heart are often at odds. These people use upper-chakra energy to muscle over the pain. They step into the courthouse and say, "My child, you need to forgive and forget," but their lower chakras still carry a lot of grief. Upper-chakra faculties never have to deal with real pain and messiness.

All healing happens through the Heart Chakra when it is in the light side, in the energy that beholds us unconditionally. It knows we are constantly evolving and accepts us for it. Heart Chakra energy flows with wisdom, like a wise, passionate, omniscient judge who sees *all* painful past events in their complete context, including all the factors involved—who we were at that point, the pressures we were under, what we did wrong and why—and everything that we also did right. We see the beautiful big picture for what it is. We see our four-year-old self at our dance recital and are filled with joy because we can appreciate the context and the unfolding. We missed almost every step and turn, but we sure tried hard. Most important, the light side of the heart knows the price we paid to learn hard lessons. This is in sharp contrast to the dark side of the Heart Chakra, which we've learned is scrutinizing and always expects perfectionism.

The Heart Chakra is special. Yet so many of us, even those who appear madly loving on the outside, are walking around with empty hearts. Before we can feel our Heart Chakra power, we need to clean house. We need to voice old wounds—our buried, personal pockets of grief—that have been preventing us from fully loving and accepting ourselves and others and blocking us from owning some crucial energy. And we need to do some forgiving. But because our rational mind tells us there is no point to unearthing our grief, we need a guide to navigate the journey. The guide for our journey into the heart is the Four Levels of Forgiveness.

In the fourth chakra we're going to walk through the Four Levels of Forgiveness. We're going to get messy and move through the stuck wounds and pain inflicted by others, as well as our resident inner critics so we can finally live and act with a joyful heart. The goal is to leave no stone unturned. We want to live in the joy of who we are in the moment. We want to look at ourselves and others adoringly as we fall and get back up again. Ironically, once we reach that point, we realize we've nothing to forgive.

FOUR LEVELS OF FORGIVENESS

Allowing the Heart Chakra to shine begins with forgiveness—or at least reaching a point where we can honestly say, "It doesn't matter." Through forgiveness and distance, we let go of grief and the inner critic and create what's known as the "undefended heart"—a heart that is accepting, kind, compassionate, forgiving, nonjudgmental, and barely, if at all, fazed by criticism. Through forgiveness, we open the floodgates, dissipating pent-up energy and releasing pure Heart Chakra energy for all the world to see. We love fearlessly. And we shine. To better understand forgiveness, I've whittled it down to four levels.

How many times have you said, "I let go of that a long time ago. I'm over that now," but maybe felt a twinge of resentment brewing underneath? That's what I call Level 1 forgiveness—the "time heals everything" approach. Maybe we didn't have the time or space for grief. If we had children to care for or a demanding job, we didn't use our free time to break down and cry. Many of us are proud of that. We soldier on, letting bygones be bygones. But if we were wronged, no matter how long ago, we need to grieve as if this event were a death.

Most of us rely on Level 1 "surface" forgiveness, but we're going to take it up a few notches. The forgiveness work we're going to do is more intense than most practitioners are willing to go. Level 2 forgives the secret, unforgivable wound we suffered by the person (usually a parent) who has hurt us the most. In Level 3 we take a hard look at our secret mistakes—the *I should have known betters*. In Level 4 we acknowledge and forgive our secret flaws. Specifically, we'll address weakness and anger.

The forgiveness tapping scripts throughout Part 4 may seem harsh, especially when it comes to forgiving seemingly minor trauma. But I make sure that you always feel safe. No one gets hurt here. I promise.

Forgiveness is a concrete path to experiencing our true nature. All forgiveness work is self-love work—radical self-love and acceptance. When we give up our terrifying secrets—our hidden wounds, fears, and guilt—we've nothing to hide. We don't get knocked off our center so easily. We feel delighted in ourselves. We feel a warmth and joy, and others feel it too. Great freedom comes from accepting all sides of ourselves, even the ugly, messy sides. To allow yourself to heal and to accept yourself completely and without judgment is the greatest act of self-love you can give yourself—and the world.

COMMENTARY BY DAVID RANIERE, PH.D.

When we think of the heart, we tend to confine our thoughts to its desirable aspects: the loving, accepting, and open parts of the heart that live in the light and are aligned with our cherished ideals. And we tend to think of the self-critical places in us, where we so harshly attack and reject unwanted aspects of who we are, as coming from somewhere else, where judgment and cruelness reside. Even a valuable term like "inner critic" can unwittingly reinforce this notion as it conjures the image of a judge or prosecuting attorney who lives more in our heads than in our hearts. And this metaphor resonates with us because this condemning voice inside us makes such a seemingly reasonable and compelling case that appears to have logic on its side.

Why is it important to recognize that the heartless inner critic is part of the heart? Because at its core, the inner critic is carrying emotional (heart) pain that it doesn't know how else to feel. It seeks to deny, dismiss, or reject what it cannot bear to feel. If we listen carefully to that voice when it's berating us in all its righteousness—not to the content of its words but instead to its tone—we may begin to hear a terrifying fear rising from within it, the loss of something that can never be replaced, or a helpless rage that can only destroy us.

If we can't hear anything, we can safely assume that that pain was experienced during some exquisitely vulnerable state. It hurt too much, and we took measures to no longer feel that unbearable pain. Much like a tourniquet is applied to save a life by cutting off blood flow to an extremity, so too do we sometimes survive by cutting off what we feel, sacrificing a part of who we are in order to keep going.

By recognizing that self-judgment and self-hatred mark places in the heart where unacknowledged grief has yet to be felt, we begin to establish a few vital pieces of understanding. First, emotional experience, and the ability to bear an emotional experience instead of cut ourselves off from it, plays a primary role in the healing process. Second, what might seem like the counterintuitive movement of leaning into a painful feeling instead of away from it is grounded in both science and wisdom.[2] And finally, we need both company and a containing structure that guides this process of making contact with our painful emotions so we can do it differently and feel something differently from the way we have felt it before.

The guided tapping processes that you will be led through in the following chapters are grounded in this understanding.

---

2 Various neurologists (e.g., Damasio 2000), research psychologists studying emotions and human development (e.g., Izard 1971, 1993; Tomkins 1962, 1963), and practicing psychoanalysts (e.g., Russell 2006; Buechler 2004) have asserted the centrality of emotional experience (affect) in both human experience and the change process. Gerald Stechler's (2003) seminal publication *Affect: The Heart of the Matter* captures this.

CHAPTER 14

FORGIVING THE SECRET WOUNDER

This process is designed to bring a profound level of healing to past hurtful and traumatic events by allowing you to get angry, in a safe and healing space, at those who hurt you the most. You get to say your piece. It's like finally having your day in court, where you get to list very specifically everything the other party did wrong *and* its impact on you. This means clearly and passionately voicing every hurt and every pain, and every single thing they have cost you, from the past all the way to the present.

As you, in your imaginary courthouse, confront those who hurt you, several important things happen. First, deeply repressed, suppressed, or denied anger and rage get to be moved up and out of your system. And isn't that what you deserve? You deserve to give yourself the space and permission for your anger to speak the truth about the unfairness of what happened to you. Expressing this in a safe space—sometimes for the first time—is liberating. It reminds us that we did not deserve what happened. Comprehending that is key to opening the Heart Chakra to your sacred deserving.

Second, as you testify to everything that you have lost, been robbed of, suffered, and never got to have, a deep well of loss and grief, previously unknown to you, is finally heard and honored and can move up and out of your system. This brings a major shift in energy in the Heart Chakra as self-compassion comes up in a way that feels profoundly warm and important. This is the experience of feeling (instead of thinking) how deserving we have always been.

Third, as you mentally take note of the intensity of all you are suddenly feeling and expressing, you get some clarity about what you really want, from how you want to be treated to the things and experiences you want in life. You sense a life-altering shift, a freedom from the past, as you take back your power and unleash a whole new, bigger rising energy that follows the release of deep anger and grief.

How Does Level 2 Forgiveness Work?

Tapping facilitates letting go of a deeper, truer lower-chakra reaction to a painful past event. It allows hurt, shock, anger, rage, vengefulness, hatred, righteous judgment, sadness, loss, and grief to be voiced, heard, and honored.

What Is the Experience Like?

The process will at times feel amazing, empowering, and validating, even though it is also intense, and at other times wrenching and draining. The is the process to move and sacredly honor stores of pain and bring a level of healing that is unprecedented for most people. You will start to understand that uncried tears and trapped anger are *supposed* to rise and be released so you can create or be called to something new in life.

Results

You will emerge unburdened, freed from the massive drain of energy it took to hold your grief. Your nervous system will be calm and nonreactive. The past event is less important to the present moment. You'll have a more fully embodied and integrated spiritual perspective over the timeline of the event in your life, including the gifts that emerged from it.

THE BIG AND LITTLE HURTS

When I talk about healing hurt and trauma, I'm referring to all levels of trauma. Trauma can result from physical, sexual, emotional, or verbal abuse. Or it can be what you might consider to be less serious—events or beliefs that impacted feelings of safety, value, worth, and lovability, such as growing up feeling somehow different from your peers. As far as we're concerned, on an energy level, trauma is trauma. No matter how major or minor it appears on the surface, trauma is devastating because it deflates our sense of power. It steals our energy and dims our light. In the tapping exercises in this chapter, we will focus on reclaiming that power.

Eventually you'll want to heal from all relationships that have caused you pain. But to start, one of the most important healings you can do is honor painful childhood experiences that resulted from your parents' limitations or choices. For the majority of people, the person who wounded them the most is a parent. Even people who grew up in what would be considered a healthy home environment have tribal wounds to address. Admitting this can be difficult for several reasons.

First, your parents may have been very sympathetic characters who actually did their best but still wounded you. If this is you, you may need to repeat the exercises until you are able to voice your version of how you were limited or what was missing. You might spend time grieving over how your parents suffered before you get to the forgiveness work. That's okay. There's no set timeline here. Everyone goes through this process in their own unique way.

Another complicating factor is that as an adult, you have adult knowledge of what made your parents the way they are, and you may feel compassion for them. That, coupled with the naturally wired and very emotional loyalty most people have toward parents, means you may resist getting angry at them, even if only in your head. It can feel like the greatest betrayal.

Leaning into Anger

Some people go through a lifetime of refusing to blatantly voice anger and blame. If you had a parent who was outwardly or explosively angry, and you experienced anger as a terrible, scary use of power, the thought of going there yourself won't make sense and might even trigger anxiety at first. Maybe you don't want to get angry at your parents because they had their own pain to deal with. Yet all of us have rage, fear, and grief underneath our wounds. When we deny it, our energy remains blocked.

Let's take the courtroom analogy again to shed some light on this. Imagine that, to pay your medical bills, you are suing someone who willfully injured you, but you refuse to testify on your own behalf. Instead you do your best to smile, look totally positive, healthy, and strong (despite the year of pain you spent in the hospital and in physical therapy) because you don't want to be a complainer. How can the judge and jury complete the process if they have not heard the whole story—*your* side of the story? They will likely make a snap decision that lacks compassion and understanding. To truly open your inner judge—your Heart Chakra—you need to let the old pain speak once and for all.

If you feel more sadness than anger, know that sadness can be sandwiched between anger and rage. Try leaning into it. In the safe space created by visualization and tapping, I encourage you to lean into sadness until you start to feel something more. Maybe it was unfair. Maybe there's someone to blame—even if it's God. Notice what feels true to you. Don't judge it. Just allow it to be voiced and see what happens.

Lastly, while you may admit that your parents screwed up royally, you may feel so angry and wounded by them that you resist giving up your anger. After all, that means going along with the story that your parents did nothing wrong, and that would not be just. The stubborn rebel inside you (no matter how much it keeps defeating you) doesn't want to let your parents off the hook. Yet this process honors of all that hurt. It allows the hurt sides to voice their truth.

At the end of the day, you don't actually have to forgive your parents. The goal is to get to a place where you honestly feel that it doesn't matter anymore. When you can achieve that distance, you've shifted the energy in your favor.

Many of you have spent your entire adult lives still in some battle with your parents. You continue to wish they could be different or wake up and change. You want your parents to admit to and apologize for all the mistakes they made and to validate you and all your wounds and gifts and choices. These battles can go on beyond the grave, long after parents have died.

So we begin Level 2 forgiveness work with this wounding story. In this exercise you'll be voicing anger, hurt, grief, or rage. This may feel completely foreign. Most people have never expressed these feelings directly to someone, particularly toward a parent they feel loyal to. But tapping is an incredible (and completely safe) facilitator of this process.

HEALING EXPERIENCE #10: LEVEL 2 FORGIVENESS

Setup Visualization #10-1

Close your eyes and take a deep breath. Allow your mind to paint a picture of your parents or caregivers as they were when you were young. Just let your mind or imagination paint that picture for you. It's okay if you think you are just remembering an old photo—just go with it.

See your parents there, and let your mind paint the picture of their limitations, their programming, their wounding, their unconsciousness, and the way that they imposed that upon you.

Now see yourself there as this beautiful light that could have shone like the sun, the beautiful, shining light of your fourth chakra, with all of your gifts and power.

Let your mind paint the picture of how that was limited because of the family, the rules, the setup, and your parents' inability to see you for the shining light you were, to honor you, to adore you.

Maybe they were loving, safe parents—but see past that for what was missing or hurtful. Because you *are* carrying some anxiety or insecurity or habitual way of operating that allowed you to adapt to not being able to be fully you.

Maybe they imposed these rules and standards about what girls could do versus boys, or maybe they had judgments or criticisms about how smart you were or weren't, or about what it meant to be weak or strong. Or maybe one or both were angry and mean and seriously damaged your self-esteem. Or maybe they played helpless and manipulated you from their victimhood, from their wounds, and they made you be the adult and that forced you to be something you weren't or something you weren't ready to be. Maybe in response you tried to be perfectly good, selfless, smart, or just invisible.

None of us is ready to be a perfect achiever or totally selfless and giving when we're only a child. So see that and get a sense for yourself of where they really robbed you. Where did they rob something from you or not allow you to be some brilliant, beautiful, amazing aspect of you? How were you limited? Maybe you were told that what you were doing was wrong, or you were told to be quiet and hide it, or you were told you had to be someone else.

We're going to start tapping about this picture. Know that you can modify the words to fit your situation more closely. You're going to tap from two perspectives—first from you as a child. This is going to be kind of weird. You'll be talking for the child that you're looking at and then switch to speaking for yourself as an adult, but you'll get the hang of it.

Tapping Script #10-1

Here I am in this house – And there's so much limitation – So much fear – So much limitation – So many rules – I have to do things a certain way, and they keep telling me things – That at a deep level – I want to resist – Things about myself – My power – My brilliance – And what I'm capable of – They're limiting me – They're controlling me – They're not keeping me safe – There's a threat there – A threat that's always there – That if I step outside of what they want, I'll be punished – I'll be chastised – I'll be disapproved of – Or maybe I'll be attacked or hit – Or I'll be ignored – I'll be abandoned – This constant threat of punishment.

Maybe they did as much right as they could – But I'm just going to honor right now – That they wronged me! – They hurt me! – They limited me! – They tore me down! – They didn't keep me safe – They didn't let me shine – They were uncomfortable with my power – And they shut it down – They told me to follow the rules – And the rules were arbitrary – The rules were based on their limitations, their paradigm – But I had to follow – And I'm still angry about it! – They never really saw me – They never really got it – And it hurts in my inner child – Sadness – Anger – Frustration – Powerlessness – Turning back to anger – My inner child frozen in this battle – Staying loyal out of fear – Doing it the right way out of fear – Doing it their way always out of fear – Fear of punishment – Abuse – Abandonment – Disapproval – Limiting myself – I learned it so long ago – Out of fear – I'm just going to honor this whole picture – And the inner child that I can see here – This was unfair, and I have the right to voice it.

Take a deep breath.

Post-Tapping Visualization #10-1

Take a deep breath. Close your eyes and see the young child that you were, again in the same situation, being limited. After tapping like that, the child in the picture will often look better and seem a little calmer or feel heard. It will be as if the child you're visualizing is saying, *Wow! They see me! They get it!* If the child is still very upset, tap through the entire script again before moving on to the next step.

Setup Visualization #10-2

Imagine that you are stepping back in time into the picture with this young child and your young parents. Now you're the protector. You're an adult, and you're there to advocate for this child. And you are going to have your day in court with the parents. Try shouting this section, even if it feels strange or like you are playacting. It will help activate and move more energy.

Tapping Script #10-2

How dare you! – You tortured me! – You hurt me – You made me feel like I was nothing sometimes – You made me feel unsafe – You made me feel unloved – Unwanted – You made me feel like who I was . . . was not enough – Broken – Bad – You really screwed me up! – And you don't even get it! – How dare you! – I'm still so angry – And you still don't see me – You still don't accept me – You still don't let me be me – And I am still in a battle with you about this – Why couldn't you do it better? – Why couldn't you figure it out? – Why were you so screwed up? – I'm so angry and hurt about it – And I never really get to voice that – So I'm honoring it today – Because I'm still in battle with you.

How dare you not see me, not honor my choices, not validate who I am! I still want you to validate me! – And I'm still struggling with the limits you gave me – I'm still struggling with the programming you gave me – And it's so wrong – It has screwed me! – I can still barely own my power – And I blame it on you – This is what you did to me, Mom and Dad – This is what you did to me – I blame you – It is all your fault – I still can't own my power because of you – I'm still in battle – Limiting myself – Rebelling – Trying to prove you wrong – And trying to get even – And trying to be loyal – And trying to win your approval – It's all happening in me – It's exhausting – And I completely blame you for every one of my problems – And that kind of feels good! – I honor this battle within me that rages on, even though I'm all grown up – I honor the energy it's taking and the distraction that it is – I'm going to honor it because here's real pain and real hurt – And I deserve to be honored – I honor myself now – And I'm open to breathing out some of this battle, some of this wounding – In a way that totally honors me.

Take a deep breath.

Post-Tapping Visualization #10-2

Close your eyes and visualize the picture again. See your parents again after that whole diatribe. Notice what your energy feels like.

This Doesn't Feel Right

If you feel guilty for saying all those negative things about your parents, that's okay.

That's just your higher self coming in really quickly as a judge and critic saying, "It's not okay for you to have your feelings if they sound mean." What we're doing is voicing the pure reaction of the second chakra to being wronged, which means reactionary anger, vengeance, blaming, and a desire to get even by saying to people, "See what you did to me?"

If you don't allow that second-chakra energy to speak and love yourself for it—to love yourself even with those feelings—then you never actually let the energy move.

Is it okay for you to have your real feelings that arise from a situation, or do you have to judge them immediately and say, "It's not okay to be mad at my parents because they did their best"? Is it okay for you to do that, to voice that and to tap? I'll answer for you: yes, it is.

Allow yourself to have the real, human feelings that arise in reaction to what happened to you, because when you voice them, you let that energy move. When feelings are not voiced, they stay locked and shoved down, and you are then locked in battle. That's how a seventy-five-year-old person can still be arguing with his long-deceased parents. He's still trying to prove something, still trying to be validated, and still trying to be loyal to a paradigm. Voice, honor, and move this energy, so you can be free of it. If guilt is coming up very strong for you, you can redo the tapping by starting with the phrase, "Even though I feel guilty saying these things, I am willing to give myself a small space to express my real hurt." That should help!

If you had an intense or violent childhood, repeat the tapping script and visualizations again and again until you start to feel calmer and see your parents become more and more distant. Typically, as the tapping progresses, compassion will arise in you—mostly for yourself but sometimes for your parents and the whole situation as well. It will feel a little less important for you to be in battle with your parents. You will feel more neutral. You won't feel as strongly about needing them to validate your choices or honor how they wronged you.

Setup Visualization #10-3

Close your eyes again and picture your parents. Picture the younger parents from the old picture of when you were a child. Next to them picture your parents of today. If your parents have passed on, just use the memory of when you last saw them. They can even be in ghostly form, because we can still argue with them even if they've passed on. We'll still hear their voices in our head. We'll think, *Oh, that was my mother's saying, and now I say it to myself.*

We're going to start tapping while imagining that we're talking to both sets of parents.

Tapping Script #10-3

I hope you've learned your lesson – I hope you've finally seen all the ways that you've wronged me and limited me and made me limit my power – I hope you've seen all the problems I've had up until now because of the way you treated me – And I'm demanding that you change – I do not accept you the way you are – Unconscious, dispassionate – Confused, mean – Selfish – I don't accept you that way – I do not accept you with your wounding and baggage – I demand you change for me – I demand you become the parents that I should have had – I demand that you apologize for everything and fix yourselves – I want you to evolve right now – And finally be the parents that I always wanted – I do not accept you the way you are – I judge it – I refuse it – And I insist that you change for me.

Be the parents that I wanted and needed right now – I want you to be loving and evolved – I want you to really see me and support me – I want you to be amazed by all the things I'm doing – And support me – I want you to change for me right now! – I refuse to accept you as you are – And I insist that you accept me – All of my light and dark – I insist that you love and accept me as I am and I'm never going to let this go – I want you to see me – And validate me – And get it! – I want you to change – I want you to be healthier – I want you to be more evolved – I want to see you be happier – I cannot accept you the way you are – But I demand you accept me!

Take a deep breath.

You just voiced something pretty honestly. And it's quite eye-opening when you realize that you are still trying to get something from your parents that is impossible to get. This keeps you locked in a battle with your parents that can never be resolved. And being in battle—even in secret—is draining because you can't change your parents or the past. But you can heal this by meeting the need you still have to be heard and validated and supported around this. This healing comes through voicing and honoring your pain, anger, and grief with compassion, patience, and understanding. You can know that what happened was wrong and that you didn't deserve it. You can know that you are and always have been good enough, lovable, and special. You can listen to what unmet need is still there but in an adult version so you can start asking for that need to be met and allowing others to give you what you need. This is how the past is healed in the present moment.

Post-Tapping Visualization #10-3

Take a deep breath and honor yourself for this moment of extreme, radical honesty. Picture your parents again and notice how you've shifted. After such a powerful tapping session, even if it only felt 50 percent true, you might experience what author Eckhart Tolle calls "extreme presence"—living completely in the present moment and feeling only compassion.

As you look back at your parents now, notice how much of your energy has been pulled back to you, into your field. Notice how you're not projecting so much energy at them anymore because it feels less important to who you are right now. All of the energy that has been circulating psychically, energetically, and unconsciously releases because you honestly voiced your wounds and tapped.

Do you need your parents to be something different so you can be seen on this planet? Or do you now have a willingness to accept them for who they are?

Looking at them now, how does your energy feel and how do your parents appear to you? As the tapping progresses, they will start to look calmer, less irrational and triggering, or sadder and more distant from your present life. And that signals progress. How much more in control and independent do you now feel about your choices and your life? Really get a sense of how much energy used to go into that battle and those unmet needs and let some self-compassion about that fill you.

I'm Still Enmeshed

If you're currently in a real ongoing battle with your living parents, or if they have a strong, controlling influence over you, tap for another hour or even daily. Some parents, particularly in certain ethnic groups, are the dominating force even over adult children. If your parents are funding you with money, that creates a whole other level of enmeshment. That's okay. Just tap as needed and notice how your relationship with your parents evolves.

Setup Visualization #10-4

Envision your parents as you saw them at the end of the last script.

Tapping Script #10-4

There they are – With all their problems – And all their wounding – And all their defenses – That comes from their life – And their experiences – And their wounding – I'm just going to let them be over there – In their energy – And their karma – On their souls' journeys – I'm going to be over here – Way over here – In my beautiful energy – Honoring myself – And honoring every living creature on this planet and where they're at – If I need to set a boundary, I can, from my powerful, beautiful energy.

Take a deep breath.

That little process of saying, "I'm going to let them be over there in their wounding, their life, and their issues that have nothing to do with me. I'm going to be over here in my energy," will create an energetic space between you and them. In doing this you pull back your energy that was in the field between you and your parents.

That, I believe, is why the next time you see your parents (or whomever you tap over), they may be and act completely differently. It's as if all the judgment and vitriol that you felt—everything you've been holding back—is suddenly released from the field between you. I don't care how "unconscious" you may think they are; they will unconsciously sense an energetic shift, and they will suddenly act differently around you.

Level 2 forgiveness is a really powerful process. I encourage you to do more of this work because it is an incredibly effective way to pull down walls and patterns and clear years of built-up issues, and it leads to a much greater experience of connection.

NEXT STEPS . . .

Your exercise this week is to make a list of at least three people in your life whom you feel overtly distressed about, or feel even an underlying level of annoyance or resentfulness about, so you can do more Level 2 forgiveness tapping.

Visit www.unblockedbook.com/chapter14 for an extra tapping experience and discussion to enhance this chapter.

CHAPTER 15

FORGIVING THE SECRET MISTAKE

We all make mistakes, but what happens afterward is important. For some small mistakes, it can be easy to take the lesson and chalk it up to learning. But what about big mistakes that really set us back? What about when we fail at something we really wanted to do well or expected to do well? A big mistake can sting for years or even a lifetime, hanging over us like a dark cloud of "evidence."

Some mistakes are traumatizing not just because of how painful they were to experience but because they change how we see ourselves. We're less likely to trust our instincts, abilities, ideas, and judgment, as if history has schooled us to believe that we're going to miss the mark again.

Then there are the events we don't call mistakes but that are just as damaging to our self-esteem, confidence, and sense of deserving. These are the times when the mistake was less about something we did and more about what we didn't do. These are the unforgivable past events. These are the times where we look back and say, "The truth is, I should have done it better."

I find that most people have no idea that holding on to past events is a problem. They feel completely right about their judgment. They don't think of these mistakes as something they have to forgive themselves for but use them as proof that they need to work harder before they deserve good things. But the bottom line is always that what they didn't know at the time, where they fell short, is in retrospect a crime that can never be atoned for. It sits in their system as unforgivable.

Holding on to something in the past that still feels totally unforgivable generates long-term damage. Every day you use some of your powerful energy to attract, manifest, and unconsciously create struggle and punishment. After all, someone who's unforgivable needs to be punished and taught a lesson. *Unforgivable* means it's not over. There's been no compensation paid or undoing of the wrong to make it right. No. *Unforgivable* means it's not over. You haven't served your time, and you still deserve to be punished.

This ongoing cycle of inner punishment turns life into a constant struggle. It shows up in little irritating ways and in broader life patterns, like never really being able to take a vacation, always feeling anxiety or guilt, or never feeling good. One client described it this way: "Margaret, I work a punishing schedule, and there is just no time for me, ever." That's the lesson being played out, manifesting in reality a life that can feel as if we were being singled out and punished.

But there are big implications to this when it comes to moving forward in life. If any mistake, misstep, or imperfect action becomes another life sentence of *Shoulda known better* or *See, I proved it again—I am not good enough,* how can we ever step outside of our comfort zone? How can we do things that we have never done before if bitter, uncompromising self-criticism is waiting on the other side? How can we tolerate the risk of bold action when secretly the stakes are so high and painful?

Level 3 forgiveness is incredibly powerful work because it has an immediate impact on how you feel in the present moment about whether you deserve good things. You can almost feel the universe shift the moment you move into your powerful Heart Chakra energy that screams, *I am so deserving right now!* When you start to live from your wise, compassionate heart, you become the loving, encouraging coach or mentor to yourself. Instead of a brutal inner critic that remembers every mistake, you have the compassion and wisdom to cheer every bit of progress, especially when doing new things, and still note where you can improve.

In this Healing Experience, the heart-opening shifts you will experience might take you by surprise, especially if you have a very active inner critic and super-high standards for yourself. Stay with it. I will continue to guide you through to the other side.

Heart-Centered People

Some of the most amazing heart-centered people who have been reading and studying about the nature of forgiveness and the heart have told me that they have never touched this level of self-compassion. That was when I realized how much of a blind spot this level of forgiveness work is, especially for people who are advanced in their study of personal growth or spirituality. We can speak about it eloquently and guide other people into self-love but feel something is missing for ourselves. This can include therapists, advanced seekers, and personal development coaches, authors, and speakers who even in their loving endeavors are still walking around being incredibly hard on themselves.

HEALING EXPERIENCE #11: LEVEL 3 FORGIVENESS

Setup Visualization #11-1

To start this Healing Experience, bring to mind a past situation that did not go well. Pick an event that, when you look back on what you did, you feel these assessments very strongly: *I should have known better. I should have been stronger. I should have been smarter. I should have seen it coming.*

It's tempting to want to take a difficult event off the table and replace it with something easier to address. If you find yourself doing this, the reason you want to avoid it may very well be because you truly feel that you are right about it—you should have known better—so there's no reason to work on it. This is exactly the right situation for this process.

To get started close your eyes and imagine this past event in which you should have known better as if it were a documentary film playing on the screen of your mind. See yourself at the part of the movie when you are making those big mistakes because you weren't "smart" enough or "strong" enough, or you didn't see it coming. See yourself actively making the mistake. For some people there is an additional difficult aspect to this story. They tell me, "Margaret, the problem is I had a feeling and I didn't listen to it. I knew there was something wrong, and I kept going." If this is true for you, notice that and be aware of it as you move into the tapping.

See that version of yourself in the movie and notice how you feel about seeing yourself actively engaged in making a huge mistake. What's the judgment you hear in your head? *I should have known better, I should have been stronger,* or *I should have been smarter*? During the tapping, you can change the wording to emphasize the judgment that fits best.

Let's jump in and start tapping.

Tapping Script #11-1

There I am – Making all the mistakes – Doing it wrong – Ugh, I still hate seeing it – Remembering all the things I didn't do right – There I am – Frozen in time in this movie – And I hate this version of me – I hate who I was being – It's painful to see myself like that – Nauseating to see myself there – But there I am – Ugh! – I should have done it better – And that is just the truth – I should have known better – I should have been stronger – And I didn't and wasn't – It is so obvious now – So clear and obvious – What I should have done – How I should have acted – And maybe I knew better – But I just kept going – There I am – So unforgivable – So unforgivable – And I am right about that – And I'll always be right – It is just the truth – And it is unforgivable – And I am never letting this go – Never – I should have known better – I should have been so much stronger – I should have known better – What was wrong with me? – I hate what I did, and I am right about that – Of course I am – It is the truth.

Take a breath.

This tapping round was more of an analysis of the facts, but there are more layers to this. If you were being really honest, what you would you say about someone who made a mistake like that? I find most people have some pretty strong feelings about that, so tune back into the movie of yourself again and finish this sentence: *The truth is I was so* _______ .

Let's jump right back in and tap on what comes next.

Tapping Script #11-2

The truth is – I was so stupid – What an idiot! – I was weak and stupid – I was clueless – It is so obvious – And so hard to look at – The stupidity – The weakness – So clueless and naive – What was wrong with me? – So upsetting to look at it – I was so unconscious – If this version of me stepped into this room – I would say, "I hate you – You idiot! – I hate what you did – You cost me everything – I'm never forgiving you" – This younger version of me – Frozen in time in this movie – Ugh! – So stupid – So unacceptable – So weak – I do not forgive this part of me – I will never let this go – Why should I? – It still hurts – I'm still angry – And I'm still paying the price – And so is everyone else – Maybe people I love still suffer – It kills me – I should have known better – I should have known better – I do not forgive myself – Not this version of me – Totally unconscious – So many things wrong – Stupid idiot! – Weak and clueless – I am still so angry, and I should be – This is truly unforgivable.

Take a breath.

Those were pretty intense words, so notice how that made you feel and what it feels like in your body. If these words still sound true, tap through both rounds again. I have had people need to tap on this 10 times before they start to feel anything move. You've been holding on to this judgment and these intensely harsh words for a long time. People with a strong willpower can stubbornly use their will to keep this punishing self-criticism going.

Eventually saying these words while tapping will create an emotional breakthrough, usually in the form of sadness and tears. See if you can feel into your Heart Chakra and notice that it doesn't feel good to be this hard on yourself. It hurts your heart every time you do it.

When the Heart Chakra opens, you will experience a rush of feeling in your heart that can be uncomfortable. This is how it feels to come out of the inner critic in our mind and feel what is happening in the heart during that criticism. Pain, sadness, grief, and tears are what *really* happens inside every time you are ruthlessly hard and dispassionate with yourself. So if you are starting to feel that shift into sadness, recognize there has been a loss of some kind that needs to be grieved.

Setup Visualization #11-3

See yourself again. Close your eyes. Visualize yourself in this image, in this movie. It may look better now, and you may have some perspective about the event. But now I want you to go back to the moment when you are still making the mistakes. See that moment again. What do you see now? How does it appear to you? Do you feel a little more compassion?

If it's still even somewhat unforgiveable, tap through the following script.

Tapping Script #11-3

There I am – And it's really hard to let this go – Because the cost was too high – It's too bad – And it wasn't necessary – It could have all been avoided – If I had just not been so stupid – If I had made a different decision – If I had just been stronger – Or smarter – Or both – Why did I not do it differently? – If I had made a better choice – It's so hard to let this go – It's like if I let it go – I have to accept it – And it's hard to accept this – It cost me so much – And it is still costing me – How can I just let this go? – When it's still costing me? – And no one really gets it – No one really understands – How much I lost that day – I lost so much – And it still hurts – I lost a lot of things – Maybe even money or a relationship – But I also lost me – I lost my confidence – Because every day since then – I don't trust myself as much – I don't like myself as much – And I do punish myself secretly about it – So I have also lost joy – The right to be happy – Because I am still paying the price – I totally honor – Everything I lost – And all the uncried tears – The grief that I don't let myself feel – Because I keep saying it is all my fault – I am just going to honor how hard that is.

Take a breath.

Honor that this is *hard* work. You may need to do a lot of tapping and reflecting as there can be a lot of layers. Tapping lets you voice the part of you that really doesn't want to forgive. It is difficult to forgive when the cost has been high, yet that grief has never been lovingly heard and held. So the process can be slow and need time and space and lots of tapping, but that is how this powerful energy will move and you will heal.

Post-Tapping Visualization #11-3

Come back to the picture and see yourself there. You might feel a little bit more compassion and even a little lighter. Now I want you to fast-forward the movie to a later time when it really hit you—when you first realized that it was all going badly. See yourself in a moment, maybe when you were alone feeling the failure, the disappointment, and the shock of how things were turning out. Maybe you are frozen with anguish on your face or weeping or trying to hold it together. See yourself there and see the pain.

Now widen your view and take stock of everything else that was going on in your life at the time—all the other pressures, people, and who you were, or your level of growth at that time. Is there any way you could have known better? Is there any way at that time, given everything else happening and the other people involved, that you could have been stronger or smarter or "seen it coming"? Or were you doing the best you knew how at the time?

Fast-forward the movie and see the painful costs ripple through time up until today. See all the costs. Not just the external ones but all the moments since that event that you have thought about it, replayed it, beat yourself up over it, and beat yourself down because of your role in it. What has holding on to the mistake cost you? What has it robbed you of and for how many years?

See yourself with the wisdom, compassion, and understanding of the heart and consider this question: Have you suffered enough yet? Have you suffered enough yet, or do you need five more years of ruthless *It's all my fault; I was an idiot* punishment? Or are you ready to heal this, let it go, and allow yourself to be happy, confident, and deserving again?

There was a price for making a mistake, and you have lived through the pain and the punishment and the consequences already. If you could step into that movie, would you really walk up to that younger version of you and say, "You deserve all this pain, and by the way, you should never forgive yourself on top of it! Yes, on top of whatever anguish you're feeling right now, I sentence you to many more years of self-punishment."

Is that what you would say? Or would you put your arm around yourself like a wise elder and be supportive?

Feel that emotion. Feel what it is like to live enveloped by a deep compassion for yourself—the compassion and understanding you deserve.

Sometimes when they do this process, people feel as if they could cry a river of tears. The sadness means that every time you say some mistake you made or some part of you is unforgivable, you break your heart and it hurts. But could you ever imagine being that hard on someone else?

There are two more things to consider about Level 3 forgiveness: Did you learn anything or take away any lessons from that event? Did surviving that event make you stronger and smarter or more aware?

THE ART OF LOVING YOURSELF

If you have already suffered enough and you got the lesson—you gained wisdom—it is time to give yourself the most amazing gift by saying, "Actually, I deserve love and good things right now! Not someday but right now! And I'm giving myself exuberant love—even though I have made mistakes."

Feel your Heart Chakra. What would it mean to be twice as loving and compassionate to yourself? To think about yourself and bubble up with joy and exuberance and a deeply felt knowing of how deserving you are of self-love and acceptance.

What would it be like if you allowed yourself to be twice as delighted with yourself? Twice as tolerant when you made mistakes? What new things could you do more fearlessly when your heart lets you be more compassionate, understanding, and patient with yourself?

Feel into your whole body, all the way down to your toes and back up to the top of your head. Feel your first chakra, your physical body, and all the tribal rules that say what's lovable and what's not. Just love it all. And your second chakra, with all your feelings and impulses—those wants and desires that are all over the map from silly to serious. And your third chakra, with your bold and authentic action and power, radiating like the sun.

Just love yourself at all those levels. Let your heart—that beautiful green Heart Chakra—radiate downward and illuminate all those aspects of yourself. Love yourself the way you love a toddler—tantrums, giggles, and all—smiling at yourself because you are adorable!

Wisdom sits in your heart. Criticism runs the show in the mind. Wisdom knows how you're integrated and has the patience to remember you are always growing and evolving. It understands that you'll always be capable of making mistakes and learning from them and giving yourself opportunities to generate even more self-love and self-compassion.

More than anything, I want you, in this moment, to exuberantly, laughingly, joyfully, and giddily love yourself. And be able to say to somebody, "I really love being me." That's what I want for you: "I love being me." When you love being you, you ask for things much more quickly and let them in because you *know* you are deserving. You ask for compassion, support, a hug, forgiveness, or an explanation.

You also ask for support and care much more quickly because you don't want to suffer or suffer alone. Not wanting punishment changes everything and everyone you are manifesting in your life. As a matter of fact, expect people who love you more than you thought you could ever be loved to start showing up in your life.

And if you think you are already loving, get ready! Doing this self-forgiveness work, which is really self-love, expands your Heart Chakra with an almost overwhelming rising love and joy for other people. It's a lot and you will feel it. Expect, as my many clients have experienced, to be moved to tears, express emotions, get and give hugs and compliments, and just simply feel life and love a lot more often. Sometimes it may feel as if you will burst! This is what I want for you!

NEXT STEPS . . .

First, think of at least one person you love and who also loves you. Picture them shining their smile at you. You can see the delight in their eyes. Picture them saying, "You're so awesome!" See how delighted they are with you. Isn't that awesome? Feel your own delight. And add some more faces of other people in your life. Feel that rising delight, the joy that rises in your heart when you think of them and hold all that in your heart and in your body until you think you might burst.

Second, be curious about when you are being impatient with yourself. Does it happen when you are scared or tired or make mistakes? Impatience is a telltale sign of inner criticisms and self-judgments that sit like little pockets just below the surface. Commit to clearing these out as you find them, and you will fill yourself with more and more joyful Heart Chakra energy.

Visit www.unblockedbook.com/chapter15 for an extra tapping experience and discussion to enhance this chapter.

CHAPTER 16

FORGIVING THE SECRET FLAW

This final Healing Experience takes you to the ultimate destination—a space of growing in self-love, acceptance, compassion, and wholeness through the deepest level of self-forgiveness. Level 4 forgiveness work uncovers and heals the secret ways in which we hate and reject aspects of our first, second, and third chakras because we learned that they are flawed, unacceptable, and broken. The two biggest, most counterintuitive aspects of this work are the qualities of weakness and arrogance, so that's what we're going to focus on.

This forgiveness work is inspired by author Debbie Ford's exploration of what she calls "the shadow side" of our nature. This is a part of our personality that we refuse to see. We reject it because we don't identify with it; it contains qualities we do not want to have. Everyone has a shadow side. The problem is finding the aspects in our shadow so we can heal, love, and integrate them into our wholeness.

In her book *The Dark Side of the Light Chasers,* Ford describes how to find these shadow side aspects. The first is to "meet your shadow," which is to honestly assess sides of yourself that you hate. These usually surface when under stress or afraid. The second is to "unmask the shadow" by noticing traits in other people that we hate and often judge as being unacceptable and therefore cannot own in ourselves. By bringing these flaws into the light, we can reckon with the dark side of them while using our heart's wisdom to see the huge amount of power they hold when properly acknowledged.

This final Healing Experience contains two complete sets of work to tap through: one on meeting the shadow and the other on unmasking it. It ends with a discussion of what is possible when we do the work to heal the hidden, unexpected spaces within us that hold self-rejection and self-judgment. When we have shifted to understanding, honoring, and even downright loving the aspects of ourselves we had learned to hate, we go far beyond healing. We become undefended, open, and incredibly courageous because we have nothing to hide. Imagine the possibilities.

HEALING EXPERIENCE #12: LEVEL 4 FORGIVENESS PART 1: FORGIVING YOUR HIDDEN SOFTNESS

Setup Visualization #12-1

To get started I'm going to ask you to think of a time in the recent or distant past when you were an adult and a complete mess. Maybe you were weak and needy or broken down with sadness and unable to get it together. If you're the type of person who has a strong will and is disciplined and always self-sufficient, you may have to look back on a time when you had the flu or a serious illness, because that's the only time you actually get messy.

Sometimes the physical body has a way of creating illness to stop you from being so self-sufficient. These are times when you likely felt shocked and betrayed by your body. And then there is what it makes you do. Most illnesses force you to be vulnerable, need support, and ask for and *let* other people take care of you and do things for you.

Close your eyes and visualize that time, just as if you were seeing it on a movie screen. See yourself there in that really broken, needy state and notice that you're not getting anything important done effectively or efficiently. When picturing yourself, you will be tempted to say something like, *Oh, my Lord, get it together! You're embarrassing yourself!* Does that resonate?

Now, regardless of what actually happened, imagine two more weeks play out—two more weeks in that state. Still getting nothing done. Just weak and sobbing and needy and ineffective. Now imagine a month has gone by. Yes, a whole month. Even if you had some compassion for yourself at first, by now you're starting to think that this is just ridiculous.

This extreme example shows how unsafe it feels for you to be weak, to not be useful, and to rely on someone else. It shows how much willpower you're using to keep yourself from ever being weak or needy.

We're going to jump into tapping, and the first thing that we're going to do is tap on this self-judgment.

Tapping Script #12-1

There I am – Oh, it's awful – So weak, so needy – I can't even look at it – I want to yell out – "You're embarrassing yourself – Get it together" – I can't stand looking at it – Weak, so weak and needy – It's embarrassing – "You're humiliating yourself!" – That's what I would say to this version of me – And this – "Get it together! – You're being useless! – And that is just unacceptable" – So needy it's disgusting. So weepy – Ugh – I was such a sad sack – What a loser, being honest – I totally judge it, totally judge myself – So needy – I totally reject this neediness – This weakness – I totally reject this part of me – It's unlikable – And the idea of people seeing me that way – Maybe I hid – Or maybe people did see – Humiliating – It's embarrassing – So weak and useless – A waste of time – Truly I was wasting time – Being all broken – Such a waste of time – Not efficient, not strong – Sobbing, embarrassing – I can't stand this part of me – I never want to see this part of me again – I never want to go there – I totally reject this part of me – Totally reject it – I don't want to know this part better – What if it takes over? – I would rather get rid of it – It's everything I hate – It gets in my way – It ruins everything – I totally reject it – And I am right, and I will never love it – Never honor it – It is good for nothing!

Take a breath.

Close your eyes and look at that part of you now. See if some of the judgment is lightening up. How does it look? When you've tapped through that round enough, you will start to feel some compassion for yourself.

When you notice some compassion for that version of you, consider how old this part of you really is. If this quality or how you were acting was a side of you, what age is it operating from? What is that side of you wanting, and what is it alone with? Because whatever those needs are, they are deep, and you are still alone with them.

Let's tap again.

Tapping Script #12-2

I see this side of me – And I reject it – But it's an old part – I'm so hard on it – And I don't want it to overtake me – That's so scary – It would overwhelm me – With an ocean of tears and weakness – It's too much. Too much sadness – Too much need – Too vulnerable and soft – Nobody wants that much neediness – No one wants someone that weak – That sad – It feels too painful – There is just so much sadness – Wanting and wanting and never getting – All this sadness – I am just going to honor – All the ways I've rejected and criticized – This real part of me – Told myself I can't be weak – That I don't deserve compassion – And I've hidden it – This deep, needy, scared place – I've done my best to hide it – So I've never been supported here – Even when people try, I push it away – I don't want them to see me like this – This needy, soft, vulnerable side of me – I've rejected and criticized it and hidden it – A lonely place, a lonely place – A lonely place – I don't want to be overwhelmed by it – But it has oceans of sadness – Ancient, old sadness – I don't trust anyone to see this side of me – Of course I don't – All this sadness, all of the sadness – I totally honor this side of me – I totally honor this side of me – And I'm willing to send it a little bit of love – Just a little bit.

Take a breath.

Look at this part of you and notice again what age it is operating from. You will never be happy, at least not in the way you want to be, if you cut off this side of you. This side of you has needs that come with strength and achievement. These needs allow you to be human and receive what you require, including support. Neediness is a difficult side of the second chakra, which makes it easy to harden our hearts to it when it appears in us as adults.

What needs does this part of you have that you learned were shameful? What needs does this part of you have that you learned were impossible? What needs does this part of you have that you learned were not going to be fulfilled by other people, such as your parents? What needs did you stop honoring or maybe even feeling?

Being vulnerable means being open. If you can't be vulnerable, you won't feel your needs or your emotions. And that means other people can't feel you either. They can't feel how much you care or your warmth. They may even call you cold and distant.

This Healing Experience is not about trying to become a needy or weak and dependent, broken-down person. It is about admitting to, honoring, owning, loving, and integrating these misunderstood aspects of yourself so you can hear what they have to say. They represent real needs that you have as an adult, and they always point to an area of your life that is way out of balance! When these needs are voiced, heard, and honored, they come into the light and can call you to a missing piece of your power, your joy—your life.

There's no sidestepping that need. You can't achieve around it. You can't learn around it. You can't drink around it. You can't be strong, sacrificing, and giving all the time, or you will never truly be happy.

So take a look one more time at this side of you in your mind's eye. It may still appear as a child and fill you with compassion. If so, imagine you can step into that picture, hold and love that little child, and allow them to cry in your arms and feel accepted and heard. That process could take some time, so don't rush it.

When that feels complete, reconnect with the child image and allow it to grow back up until it looks like you again. This is your adult vulnerable side that is there to remind you that you are human and at times need patience, care, understanding, and help! Picture this version of you saying, "I need help!" and notice how that feels. When we don't hear this side of us, or ever allow it to surface, we will feel as if we can never relax and that we are always on our own—even when in a loving relationship.

NEXT STEPS . . .

Keep sitting with this side of you and ask questions such as: *What does this side of me need? What does it want? What would fill it with joy, giddiness, and pleasure? What would allow this side of me to fill up with deliciousness? How deeply does it feel? How much more deeply does it feel than I let myself feel? How scared am I to let it out of the basement, and what would it mean if I started to listen to what it wants?*

Write down your answers. Make a list of what you want. Play with words such as *adored, worshipped, loved, pleasure,* and *power.* Just sit with these words, even if they are triggering. And remember: this side of you has *so much power* for you.

HEALING EXPERIENCE #12: LEVEL 4 FORGIVENESS PART 2: FORGIVING THE HIDDEN PIECE OF YOUR POWER

In this second part of Level 4 forgiveness, we will use the "unmask the shadow" process mentioned earlier to see a rejected side of our power through someone else. We will focus on another set of second-chakra traits that are usually described as arrogance and anger. Although they have negative connotations, these energies hold a huge gift for you.

Setup Visualization #12-3

Close your eyes and take a deep breath. Bring to mind someone in your life, either past or present, who is arrogant, selfish, *and* willing to be angry. Maybe it is an ex or a boss or a parent or a business partner who wronged you or betrayed you.

Imagine you are looking at that person as if they were standing in front of you, and they are at their worst. Maybe they are being loud or obnoxious and boastful or demanding and complaining. Really take them in. Notice how they look and how you feel being around them acting that way.

Many of my clients will say they really don't enjoy being around this person at all and find them difficult to tolerate. Notice how they make you feel. Are you angry, terrified, or scared? Do you feel small? Now imagine you could roll your eyes and step back a bit, observing them from a distance, and let yourself be totally judgmental. How would you describe them? What words would you use if you were being brutally honest? How does that feel in your body, looking at that person with your judgments? Notice how your judgments probably feel quite justified and on point. Notice if you find yourself saying, *I would never be like that!*

We have now unmasked this shadow in your angry and arrogant person. Let's start tapping. As we go through the script, feel free to insert words that best describe the most unacceptable or triggering qualities about them. Some examples I commonly hear are: *out of control, selfish, greedy, mean, vindictive, narcissistic, manipulative, self-absorbed, self-important, egotistical,* and *uncaring.*

Tapping Script #12-3

There they are – I can see them so clearly – So selfish – So arrogant – So angry – Out of control angry – So selfish – So mean – Hurting people – With their anger – And their selfishness – They don't care about other people – Don't care who they hurt – So selfish – Only think about themselves – I totally judge them – And I totally should – I am right about this – It's unacceptable – So angry and mean – They only care about themselves – I would never do that – And I totally judge that – And I would never be that way – It's hurtful – It is wrong and hurtful – And so arrogant – Think they are so great – Acting so grandiose – What an ego trip! – Demanding – Complaining – And so entitled – Really don't care about other people – And I care about people so much – I totally judge how selfish they are – And that awful out-of-control anger – It's unacceptable – It's scary – It's so unkind and ugly – It's so hurtful – I would never accept that – I totally judge it – I will never say that is okay – And I would never want to look like that – I would never be like that – I would never want anyone to say this about me – And I have spent my life – Making sure I never act like that – Maybe even going to great lengths – To prove I am better than that – That I am not anything like that!

Take a deep breath.

Post-Tapping Visualization #12-3

Look at that picture again. Look at the person you were picturing before and see how they look.

How do you feel now while looking at this person? Depending on the history, you may need several rounds of tapping here, especially if this person carried a lot of anger, played a part in a very painful incident, or was angry or abusive for years. It's critical to do as many rounds of tapping as necessary to fully release that charge and voice and honor all of your anger, hurt, and loss.

Once that feels complete, the picture will change. They will look smaller and calmer. Once you are there, consider this question: Although the way this person acts is obviously over-the-top negative and hurtful, what does someone who acts like that get to experience? What is the gift in the ability to be angry, arrogant, and selfish and to let people know when you think something is unfair to you?

When I have asked these questions over the years at this part of the process, these are the answers I consistently get:

What's the gift in anger? You can step up, own your power, carry a little more energy, have a bigger boundary, and ask for what you want.

What is the gift in arrogance? You truly own and believe in your value and are willing to let people know your worth.

What is the gift in selfishness? You get to set a boundary without feeling guilty because you get to put your own interests first.

What if you totally owned that an inner part of you is calling you, in certain situations, to be a little more selfish, arrogant, or even angry in a way that feels like a gift and is honoring you?

When we only see the shadow side of these qualities, it's easy to put them on others and vow to never be like them. But this cuts us off from using these energies when we need them for our highest good.

The gift that you find in answering this question is always something that you already know you need to do more of in your life! Well, guess what—a part of you wants to rise up and give you the courage and energy to own the light side of that quality. It just usually gets ejected and judged as all bad.

Let's tap.

Tapping Script #12-4

Even though I really judge this person – And they probably deserve it – I'm just going to own and honor – That I have an angry, selfish side – It is in there – I don't really like to look at it – I judge that part of me too – I love and accept myself – All of me – Even with this angry, selfish side – Even though it's really easy to see – The terrible downside of anger, arrogance, and selfishness – And I've spent a lot of time judging this person – The truth is there's a part of me – That's calling me to have a little more anger – Maybe self-advocate – To be a little more selfish – And that would actually be a gift in my life – To be a little more arrogant – And own my value – To own my hard-earned authority – In the light.

The truth is I can carry all my qualities – I can be fully dynamic – As a whole, conscious person – I can be really angry – And still be very loving and have a really big heart – I often say I'm not selfish – And I've gone to great lengths to prove it – The truth is I have a selfish side – It actually doesn't look that different – From this person's selfish side – When you boil it down – Their selfish side may be quite immature – In many ways this person is like a child – But this is about me – And I now honor all of me – The gift and the selfish, angry side – The gift of arrogance and demanding what you want – The gift of speaking up when something feels unfair – That I've always missed out on – By judging it – It's calling me to balance – Stand in my power more – Be a little more selfish – That's been way out of balance – This is actually a pretty big gift for me – It feels really different – To honor that I need to come first sometimes – Can I really honor that? – And still know that I am a loving and compassionate person? – It would feel really different to honor that I am both – It would be really different to honor the gift and calling in selfishness – It would be really different to honor the gift and calling in anger – The gift and calling in arrogance – Strange but good – I'm open to honoring all of me – My dark and my light.

Take a deep breath and notice how you feel.

This kind of work is counterintuitive and, yes, strange. Take some time to be with it and to challenge your habitual way of thinking and feeling about it. And notice over time that as you own and honor these energies for their light, you will likely be less triggered by this person and others like them. That doesn't mean they are easy to be around or that you have forgiven them; just that you find them less triggering. Instead of wondering why they act the way they do and feeling compelled to rehash their latest bad behavior with friends or in your head, you will just shrug it off. I find people are both less fazed and much more likely to deal with that person with a more grounded leadership energy that includes boundaries.

The best part of owning these qualities is that you no longer have to prove you do not possess them. I wasted years of my life doing things to prove I was not selfish, and no matter what happened, I was "bigger than getting angry." The need to *not* be selfish or angry cut my power off at the knees and had me do many things that were not in my best interest. It also made me easy to manipulate because that was my weak spot! All you had to was suggest that I was being selfish, and I would launch into more self-sacrificing and undo boundaries just to prove I was not selfish. But, of course, I was. You can't be human and not have some impulses to put yourself, your survival, your happiness, and your well-being first.

This is how we arrive at being undefended and experiencing the lightness and freedom that comes with that. When we have looked at, understood, and owned our secret fears and worrisome dark sides, what insult can crush us? What criticism or judgment can collapse our power and have us run for cover? When we acknowledge that we carry our own version of embarrassing qualities, that fact changes absolutely nothing because we still carry the light sides as well.

We can be selfish and totally generous and giving. We can be arrogant and have moments when we feel humbled to our core. It's an exhilarating freedom, like removing big red buzzer buttons that have been stuck all over your body that anyone could push at any time to stop you in your tracks.

NEXT STEPS . . .

This week, ask yourself the following questions once a day:

- How would my life look if I carried a little more power?
- What if I admitted I needed to be more arrogant, more selfish, and even more angry and demanding?
- What would owning those qualities give me the energy and courage to do?
- What would that look like, and is that the gift that I need and will need for my next chapter in life?

Visit www.unblockedbook.com/chapter16 for an extra tapping experience and discussion to enhance this chapter.

EPILOGUE

Your Next Chapter: Living the Power of All Seven Chakras

Unblocking and reclaiming empowerment energy is possible—not to mention rewarding, meaningful, and necessary to leading a full life. I've used this work on myself and thousands of clients for more than a decade. When we're able to voice, move, and release the inner problems that underlie our complaints and struggles, we are *transformed*—sometimes instantly in the relief we feel, or in a bold new action we suddenly find ourselves taking.

Now confident, passionate, and courageous, we believe in ourselves deeply as we realize that not believing in ourselves was never actually warranted. With that bitter inner critic silenced and no longer tearing us down when we make a mistake, we comprehend how deserving, amazing, and lovable we have always been. We're *on fire* and *in action.* We speak up with authority. We lead. We are enthusiastic, joyful, and memorable, and light up any room we walk into. We become our true, authentic selves—the people we were meant to be. We are unblocked, and we are empowered. We are powerful.

Unblocking this energy has positively affected my life in so many ways. I'm more alive, passionate, and connected, and fearlessly doing things I never imagined I could do. At the same time, I am kinder to myself when I am fearful, anxious, or insecure. I am both stronger and softer at the same time, putting in the effort to do big things and still making mistakes.

The more I am willing to be authentic, the more my business blossoms. I believe in myself enough to market myself boldly with willingness, enthusiasm, vulnerability, and courage. I am seen for my gifts, and I allow my heart to be more known and felt by others. And boy, it is so much easier and fun to just be myself than to try to be someone who's perfect and never makes a mistake.

THE BIGGER PICTURE

While we've been working on each of the lower four chakras in isolation and as a means to heal and charge up our empowerment energy—and you have truly been courageous—there is a bigger picture.

Doing this work is important. Not only for our own gratification but quite frankly for the world. The level of violence versus peace on the planet, for instance, will be affected by the personal work you do around fear and anger. One person enthusiastically loving and being themselves gives everyone around them permission to be imperfect and still love themselves. It's contagious. And so we become a force on this planet—a true, honest-to-goodness superhero.

When we show up fully conscious and empowered, we're positioned to positively impact people, places, and things. Decisions based on our full-body truth instead of a ragtag collection of beliefs that come from our history manifest a better world. It's the ripple effect. And it spans far and wide.

One of my greatest joys, in fact, is teaching coaches, therapists, healers, and people from every walk of life how to use this work, whether on themselves or with clients, loved ones, or communities. Expanding the ripple is now my most passionate mission.

UPPER-CHAKRA INTEGRATION

At this point in the journey, we arrive ready to recognize and use the gifts and power of the upper chakras. So it is fitting here to touch on what is now possible. By incorporating the three upper chakras into our being, we build on that bedrock of empowerment energy and start to shine as a whole person.

The upper chakras, no longer contaminated by lower-chakra hurts and misperceptions, are free to support us in quantum leaps of progress. They are critical tools, calling us to a higher purpose and vision and unimaginable possibility. For example, the seventh, or Crown, chakra gifts us with flashes of inspiration and possibility, from the small—like a radical ingredient added to a recipe—to the life-altering, such as the change of direction we see during a midlife crisis or career change.

On a practical day-to-day basis, our upper chakras serve the mission we have consciously chosen by liberating our empowerment energy. Sitting in the middle and belonging to both the upper and lower chakras, the Heart Chakra takes our passionate rising wants and readiness to act and brings wisdom and awareness of how other people will be included in and impacted by our goals and dreams. With this more mature and inclusive energy, our goals evolve from the limited lens of the "me" focus to the expansive "we" focus. This is how the pain of our personal story can drive our early goals and later evolve into a bigger, passionate mission or cause.

The powerful sixth chakra, or Third Eye, illuminates everything through a clear lens when the distortions of the lower chakras are healed. Instead of fending off danger of a worrisome future and impending disappointment, our mind's eye will seek the way, the plan, the strategy, and the necessary knowledge and resources with the clarity of single-minded focus. Instead of looking in the old distorted fun-house mirror at ourselves and others, we see a symphony of gifts, talents, and experiences that everyone brings in perfect timing and unison, where everyone has their own win-win.

When freed from automatically speaking the truth of our family, our fears, and our secret pain, the fifth chakra, the Throat Chakra, becomes the channel for true life creation. In *How to Know God*, author Deepak Chopra sums it up: "You just intend a thing and it happens." When you think about it, everything we want to do, be, and have starts with how we speak to ourselves and others about it.

THE END OF THE RAINBOW

Think of the chakra system as a rainbow—all the chakras working in concert, moving dynamically from one mode to the next to reach a goal using fully conscious energy. To illustrate this in real terms, imagine working with an outstanding boss—one person capable of easily and effectively providing whatever people need in any given moment to get the job done.

Sometimes a team needs first-chakra safety and support. If under a tight deadline to produce a product, for instance, a good boss makes sure to meet logistical and physical team needs. This might include modifying the physical workspace, requesting the right equipment, having lunch delivered, and defining laser-focused project roles and responsibilities so everyone is working in unison. The boss contains the anxiety and stress from the pressure, letting the team know they're all in this together and everyone has their role to play. Everyone feels safe and supported in the structure and culture of the team and company and clear about their next step.

Having the right resources only takes you so far. A good boss holds a second-chakra pep rally cheering everyone on and energizing employees to fearlessly go for the big win. At the point when the team needs to buckle down and do the work, the third chakra brings self-discipline, focused action, and willpower. The boss also takes note when the pressure gets too high or a setback brings discouragement and frustration and brings in fourth-chakra energy. They call for a pause with a team huddle to voice and hold an honest space for the pain in the undercurrent and allow the team to take a deep breath, reconnect, and remember why they're doing what they're doing.

The upper chakras bring clarity and direction. At the fifth chakra, the boss is in charge, decisive, and consciously directing and reaffirming the team's commitment. Sixth-chakra energy delivers clear vision and a plan for success so even when things seem uncertain, the boss is inspired and undeterred. And at the seventh chakra, the boss holds the space once or twice a year for open brainstorming, asking, "Imagine there are no barriers or limitations. What would the perfect solution look like? What is possible if we think bigger?"

Imagine all of that empowerment energy and all of those leadership qualities in one person—you. This is how chakra energy moves when it's not blocked. It's dynamic, powerful, self-reflective, compassionate, and always looking to the greater good for win-win-win-win. It's the pot of gold at the end of the rainbow.

CAPTAIN MARVEL IS YOU

One of my favorite superhero stories is depicted in the 2019 Marvel movie *Captain Marvel*. The first time I saw it I felt as if the story were about me, but it's really about all of us. In case you haven't seen it, this is a bit of a spoiler alert.

Basically, aliens capture Captain Marvel just as she acquires her massive powers. She's unconscious at the time and has no memory of how she got her powers. Because she is so incredibly powerful, the aliens want to keep and use her for their purposes. They give her a mentor who seems to care about and support her. They install a device in her neck to literally control her nervous system and shut down her power instantly (an interesting parallel to how fear and shame can so quickly shut us down). They convince her that *they* are gifting her this power and withholding some of it because she doesn't deserve all of it. She has to prove she is worthy of it, but she's not "strong enough." For most of the movie, Captain Marvel is constantly trying to prove herself worthy. (Does this resonate yet?)

Regular "proving" sessions take place as her stronger and wiser mentor challenges her in hand-to-hand combat, during which she is forbidden to use her powers. Repeatedly she is knocked down, overpowered, and put in her place, and fails the challenge. Each time he'd say something to the effect of, "See, you're still too weak. You don't deserve to have more power. You're still too weak."

As I stop here and highlight all the techniques used to limit and control her true power, I invite you to take stock of versions of these in your life. Then think bigger too, and consider how these have been used in families, religions, cultures, and workplaces:

- They purposely use a built-in weakness to instantly shut down all her strength, leaving her reeling, apologizing, and thoroughly chastised.
- She is repeatedly challenged with no-win situations—impossible tests with impossible standards to keep her busy and distracted and to reinforce the tribal agreement that she is not worthy or ready yet to hold any more power.
- She is given just enough encouragement to make her useful and feel part of the team, and to have hope that someday she will succeed and everything will be different.
- Her very memories have been "edited" so she can only recall the times when she screwed up—when she was knocked down, failing, getting in trouble, and being yelled at, injured, or humiliated. That's all she can see when she looks back on herself—someone who always failed.

Captain Marvel eventually overcomes these manufactured limitations. A key turning point is when she reconnects with her earthly tribe—the group of people who once knew, loved, and supported her. They hold up a different mirror, showing her who she was, who she is, and who she can be. They call her "captain" because she was a captain—a leader—in the armed services (which means she took an oath to serve and protect constitutional rights). This opens up something lost within her, and she begins to question the old mirror used to manipulate her. Then she starts to question everything, and that's when she gets extremely pissed off!

Like any good uprising against oppression, her rebellion is met by renewed efforts to control her. I mean, who does she think she is? But this final time, her anger and righteous outrage over how the aliens have controlled her overcomes the built-in control mechanisms. She first battles the voice in her head, and in that victory suddenly sees something mind-blowing. With the veil lifted, she finally sees the rest of the story—not just isolated memories of defeat but also the moments of strength and courage that her oppressors cut from her memory bank.

She can now see how she *got up* when she fell. Not just once but many times. She sees the part of the story when she brushed herself off and stood defiantly, even with tears in her eyes, undeterred in her fearlessness. She realizes she's failed, fallen, recovered, and overcome hundreds of times. She is not weak and unworthy! She's strong, courageous, invincible, and unstoppable!

With her inner critic now vanquished, she bursts into action in the real world, easily besting her mentor as he tries to goad her with the old mind tricks. The audience cheers as she finally blasts him with pure energy from her body and then marches up to where he lies bewildered and declares her new freedom in one stunning aha moment, saying, "I have nothing to prove to you."

We do love a hero's story, don't we? Especially in the moment when the hero truly realizes their power and mission and defeats the oppressors with flair!

Here we come full circle to you in your own hero's journey. What phase are you in, what support are you getting, and what pushback are you ready to overcome?

HEALING ON A LARGER SCALE

The personal growth in this book represents a hero's journey inside of one person—you. But as is the microcosm, so is the macrocosm. The same empowerment work, progress, and challenges you've been doing in this book are reflected in groups of people making social change.

A founding principle written in the Declaration of Independence asserts there are certain natural and legal rights, including the right to revolt. The second sentence is one of the most famous statements invoked by human rights activists and protesters for change: "We hold these truths to be self-evident, that all men are created equal, that they are endowed by their Creator with certain unalienable Rights, that among these are Life, Liberty and the pursuit of Happiness."

What happens when a group of people starts to realize that they truly do have the right to not just live but pursue freedom and happiness? What happens when a group of oppressed people starts asking for and demanding those rights, breaking long-accepted norms of a culture or society? There is always pushback, intimidation, and loud retorts, as well as innuendos insinuating that, well, you certainly do *not* have the right. That shameful *Who do you think you are?* message is powerful. Tribes seem to intuitively know how to wield its potency.

THE PUSHBACK STAGES OF EMPOWERMENT

The first phase is always the necessary building anger that turns into the courage to speak up and protest as a show of commitment to the new awakening. We have lived this painful process many times over throughout history and across the globe as societies rupture with the anger and grief that leads to slow, messy progress.

You will experience the same type of pushback in your journey too, from your family, employer, and even friends. Anticipating this pushback as you evolve and move into your next chapter gives you the upper hand, especially given that you now understand what's happening. It isn't personal. It's tribal. It's universal. And it's a stage you can get through by standing firm and up-leveling.

Are you ready to embrace the first wave of pushback? To rage and cry as you have learned to do in this book, and use your voice to assert your growing certainty of what you deserve and what you have the right to?

It would be easier if a hero's journey ended at the winning, as it does in the movies! In real life progress takes two steps forward with small steps backward. But take heart. This has always been the way of our world.

Let's look again at the macrocosm: What happens in real life when a large group of people finally wins the rights that they fought so hard for? There is celebration, recognition, and a tipping point of advancement, and then a cultural shift. But the changes come with a price, as not everyone is always on board.

I remember the happy, affirming feelings I had during the sexual harassment trainings at work that started taking place in the early nineties. Finally, we were making progress! But harassment didn't disappear. I watched the less overt but insidious way it still played out through those who grumbled about how ridiculous and unnecessary the whole thing was. "What? Now I can't say you look pretty in your dress today?"

In any revolution a percentage of people remains unconvinced and determined to keep the old way alive. For them the story is different. They may have given in for the moment, but not because they recognize and honor a true right. This is critical to understand. They see the progress as a concession that they have "gifted" or allowed. The beneficiaries of their gratuity now need to be eternally thankful. In my experience, getting a promotion as woman used to mean years of gratitude, loyalty, and being reminded of what you "owe" for this extraordinary gift.

Mika Brzezinski talks about this in her book *Know Your Value* as a common theme among women in powerful positions. They don't ask for much because they tell themselves they should be "so grateful" to have the opportunity. No one will argue with you if you never ask for a raise or equal treatment yet keep working harder. Loyalty to the tribe works for those in power.

With all our chakras working full-on, we can be both grateful and know in our bones what we want and deserve at each stage so we can ask for it. Usually this integration goes well as we progress, except when we encounter people with whom we have trouble setting boundaries.

Looking back at the macro scale, what happens when rights are won and become the norm for a while in society? That same group of people who used their second-chakra outrage to win their protest and got their first-chakra rights on paper will push past the initial celebration and take third-chakra action. This means they start openly acting as if those rights truly are their rights. When you win the right to vote, you fully expect to be able to safely show up at the polls and cast a ballot.

Acting on newly claimed rights always triggers a second wave of pushback that is often unexpected. Suddenly a social veneer erupts, revealing the simmering resentment that has been boiling in those on the other side who see this action as adding insult to injury. Now we hear the next iteration of *Who do you think you are?* Only this round includes specialized words such as *entitled, uppity, ungrateful*—words used as weapons to shame and intimidate.

These words are the old way clawing back to say you don't have the right. This was the situation after men newly emancipated from slavery were granted the right to vote in 1870, which was followed with nearly a century of Jim Crow laws and voter suppression.

I have worked with many successful women who were shocked to find themselves on the receiving end of these *Now you've gone too* far attacks from people they never expected to react this way, including spouses and co-workers. Even more common, however, is when this pushback comes from our own inner critic, the inner saboteur that lives in our head. Remember that, because now you are wide awake. You are wise and have the tools to overcome even the inner setbacks. This is up-leveling at its best.

These are the moments when we thought we'd already slayed that dragon and were done. But alas and alack, we have to dig deeper into our ever-budding self-love, self-belief, and self-worth. These are the moments when we must once again check in and reaffirm what we believe about what we deserve and what we have the right to have, to do, and to be.

These are the moments we must again feel our rising anger, outrage, and courage to stand strong, protest, and set a boundary, even if only with ourselves. These are the moments we are called to lead with conviction and humanity. To lead with leadership energy is the only way to make true change, whether in our town, country, globally, or simply within our own inner microcosm of self-empowerment.

So don't be shocked! Be wise, be powerful, and be real! Be more willing to leave no stone unturned in unblocking your power. Know the stages of empowerment and pushback chakra by chakra and do the real work each step of the way. I promise it gets light-years easier once the weight of the past is healed and lifted through the many Healing Experiences in this book.

Though you may never have Captain Marvel's laser blaster, what may seem now like an impossibly high barrier in front of you will shrink to a stepping-stone as you build on your progress and strengthen your chakra muscles. I do promise that, like a true human superhero, you will rise, you will fly, and you will be unstoppable, all while holding the world in your heart! Imagine what is possible when you do. Imagine the impact you will make and how it will feel to make it.

As Captain Marvel says as the end of her first chapter: "I've been fighting with one arm tied behind my back. . . . But what happens when I'm finally set free?"

What happens indeed!

INDEX OF TAPPING SCRIPTS AND VISUALIZATIONS

READING LIST

Banyan, Calvin. *The Secret Language of Feelings.* Richardson, Texas: Banyan Hypnosis Centre, 2002.

Brown, Brené. *Daring Greatly.* New York: Avery, 2015.

Brzezinski, Mika. *Know Your Value.* New York: Hachette, 2018.

Ford, Debbie. *The Dark Side of the Light Chasers.* New York: Riverhead, 2010.

Judith, Anodea. *Eastern Body, Western Mind.* New York: Celestial Arts, 2004.

Myss, Caroline. *Anatomy of the Spirit.* New York: Harmony, 1996.

REFERENCES

Adamson, Lauren, and Janet Frick. "The Still Face: A History of a Shared Experimental Paradigm." *Infancy* 4, no. 4 (2003): 451–473.

Bollas, Christopher. *The Shadow of the Object: Psychoanalysis of the Unthought Known*. New York: Columbia University Press, 1987.

Buechler, Sandra. *Clinical Values: Emotions that Guide Psychoanalytic Treatment*. New York: Routledge, 2004.

Brennan, Barbara. *Hands of Light: A Guide to Healing through the Human Energy Field*. New York: Bantam Books, 1987.

Damasio, Antonio. *The Feeling of What Happens: Body and Emotion in the Making of Consciousness*. New York: Harcourt, Inc., 2000.

Freud, Sigmund. *Civilization and Its Discontents*. Hogarth, 1930.

Hesse, Hermann. *Demian: The Story of Emil Sinclair's Youth*. New York: Penguin Books, 2013.

Izard, Carroll E. *The Face of Emotion*. New York: Appleton-Century-Crofts, 1971.

Izard, Carroll E. *Face of Emotion*. Irvington Publishers, 1993.

Mesman, Judi, Marinus H. van IJzendoorn, and Marian J. Bakermans-Kranenburg. "The Many Faces of the Still-Face Paradigm: A Review and Meta-Analysis." *Developmental Review*, 29, no. 2 (2009): 120–162.

Modell, Arnold. "The Origin of Certain Forms of Pre-Oedipal Guilt and the Implications for a Psychoanalytic Theory of Affects." *International Journal of Psychoanalysis*, 52, no. 4 (1971): 337–346.

Nathanson, Donald L. *Shame and Pride: Affect, Sex, and the Birth of the Self.* New York: W.W. Norton and Co., 1992.

Russell, Paul. "Trauma, Repetition, and Affect." *Contemporary Psychoanalysis*, 42, no. 4 (2006): 601–620.

Stechler, Gerald. "Affect: The Heart of the Matter." *Psychoanalytic Dialogues*, 13, no. 5 (2003): 711–726.

Tomkins, Silvan S. *Affect/Imagery/Consciousness: Volume 1: The Positive Affects*. New York: Springer, 1962.

Tomkins, Silvan S. *Affect/Imagery/Consciousness: Volume 2: The Negative Affects*. New York: Springer, 1963.

Tronick, Edward, Nadia Bruschweiler-Stern, and Alexandra Harrison. "Dyadically Expanded States of Consciousness and the Process of Therapeutic Change." *Infant Mental Health Journal*, 19, no. 3 (1998): 290–299.

Tronick, Edward, Heidelise Als, and Lauren Adamson. "The Infant's Response to Entrapment Between Contradictory Messages in Face-to-Face Interaction." *Journal of American Academy of Child Psychiatry*, 17 (1978): 1–13.

Van der Kolk, Bessel. *The Body Keeps the Score: Brain, Mind, and Body in the Healing of Trauma*. New York: Penguin Books, 2014.

INDEX

A

B

S

U

V

W

ACKNOWLEDGMENTS

First and foremost I would like to thank my husband, David, for going on this journey with me into *Unblocked*, both in writing it and in the years of helping me understand and explain my deepest work. I also want to thank my parents, Marguerite and Pete Lynch, for raising me with love, encouragement, and grounded, practical wisdom, and my brothers and sisters for their continual support mixed with hilarity.

I want to thank my business partners, Bethany Long and Beverly Carter, who have been with me almost since day one of my journey from corporate America to private coaching to training thousands of coaches and therapists in my methods. Together with my whole team, you make work fun because we are in it together!

A huge thank-you goes to Karen Chernyaev, who worked with me tirelessly in writing this book, and to my editor Melody Guy at Hay House, who brought direction and enthusiasm from day one.

I also want to thank some of my expert mentors who believed in me early on and honored me with years of help, support, and friendship, specifically Alan Davidson, Nick Ortner, Glen Ledwell, Jeff Walker, and Dawson Church. I would not be here without you, and I am so grateful! Finally, I want to honor my "Mastermind Family," who have held the loving and badass space for me to be challenged, step up, fall, and grow—I love you guys!

—Margaret Lynch Raniere

ABOUT THE AUTHORS

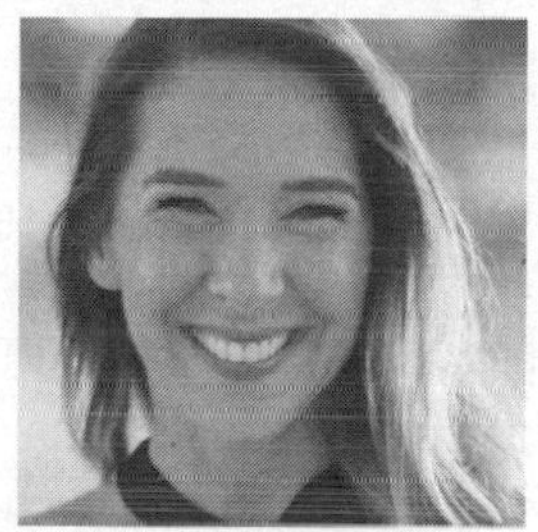

Margaret M. Lynch Raniere is an author, speaker, personal development coach and trainer, and owner and CEO of MargaretLynchRaniere.com, a million-dollar online business dedicated to sharing her unique blend of transformational healing. Over the past decade, Margaret has gained wide recognition for her cutting-edge work integrating clinically proven energy-psychology techniques with world-class teachings about the chakras to create a systematic, step-by-step, highly effective approach to healing. By combining Emotional Freedom Technique (EFT), a powerful set of unique and proprietary scripts, and chakra work, Margaret has taken chakra healing to the next level. Thousands of personal development coaches, therapists, and everyday people from all over the globe enjoy her wildly popular coaching programs and systems, live events, instructional videos, and books.

Margaret is author of the popular *Tapping Into Wealth* (Penguin/Tarcher, 2013). The *Wall Street Journal* called her "the wealth manifestation authority" because of her focus on skyrocketing wealth and impact by clearing inner blocks while building "on-fire enthusiasm and charisma."

Unlike many well-known personal development authors and speakers, Margaret's foundation is in engineering and business. She earned a bachelor of science in chemical engineering from

Worcester Polytechnic Institute, and after an 18-year career, during which she won top sales awards at Fortune 500 companies, Margaret left corporate America to live her passion: helping others transform into their most powerful selves.

Because of her engineer training, Margaret sees the chakras as a methodical approach to solving problems and getting tangible results. The chakras are a road map, a concrete pathway to healing. When used in conjunction with EFT and Margaret's powerful scripts, people experience immediate results.

Margaret has extensive certification in EFT, a clinically proven and highly effective mind-body healing tool. She is a 10-time presenter at the Tapping World Summit, an active committee member of the Association for Comprehensive Energy Psychology, and belongs to the Jeff Walker Platinum Plus Mastermind, an elite entrepreneurial mastermind for Internet marketing. She is a former member of Business Networking International.

Margaret has been featured in the *Wall Street Journal*, *Boston Globe*, *Miami Herald*, *Houston Chronicle*, and *San Francisco Chronicle*, as well as on NBC, ABC, CBS News, FOX, and CNN.

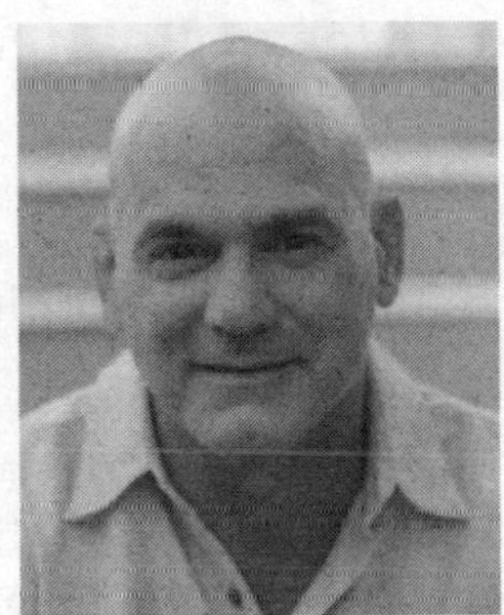

David Raniere, Ph.D., is a psychologist and psychoanalyst who uses EFT in clinical practice. He received his doctorate in clinical psychology from Temple University before completing a two-year postdoctoral fellowship at Harvard Medical School. Dr. Raniere finished his formal psychoanalytic training at the Massachusetts Institute for Psychoanalysis, where he now serves as faculty and supervising analyst. He is also adjunct faculty at William James College. Dr. Raniere has served as the clinical director and director of training at the Boston Institute for Psychotherapy and currently maintains a private practice in Framingham, Massachusetts.

Hay House Titles of Related Interest

YOU CAN HEAL YOUR LIFE, the movie,
starring Louise Hay & Friends
(available as an online streaming video)
www.hayhouse.com/louise-movie

THE SHIFT, the movie, starring Dr. Wayne W. Dyer
(available as an online streaming video)
www.hayhouse.com/the-shift-movie

***

CHARGE AND THE ENERGY BODY: The Vital Key to Healing Your Life, Your Chakras, and Your Relationships, by Anodea Judith

MENTOR TO MILLIONS: Secrets of Success in Business, Relationships, and Beyond, by Kevin Harrington and Mark Timm

MIND TO MATTER: The Astonishing Science of How Your Brain Creates Material Reality, by Dawson Church

TAPPING INTO ULTIMATE SUCCESS: How to Overcome Any Obstacle and Skyrocket Your Results, by Jack Canfield and Pamela Bruner

THE TAPPING SOLUTION: A Revolutionary System for Stress-Free Living, by Nick Ortner

All of the above are available at your local bookstore,
or may be ordered by contacting Hay House (see next page).

***

We hope you enjoyed this Hay House book. If you'd like to receive our online catalog featuring additional information on Hay House books and products, or if you'd like to find out more about the Hay Foundation, please contact:

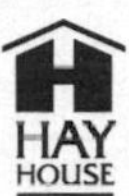

Hay House, Inc., P.O. Box 5100, Carlsbad, CA 92018-5100
(760) 431-7695 or (800) 654-5126
(760) 431-6948 (fax) or (800) 650-5115 (fax)
www.hayhouse.com® • www.hayfoundation.org

Published in Australia by: Hay House Australia Pty. Ltd., 18/36 Ralph St., Alexandria NSW 2015
Phone: 612-9669-4299 • *Fax:* 612-9669-4144
www.hayhouse.com.au

Published in the United Kingdom by: Hay House UK, Ltd., The Sixth Floor, Watson House, 54 Baker Street, London W1U 7BU
Phone: +44 (0)20 3927 7290 • *Fax:* +44 (0)20 3927 7291
www.hayhouse.co.uk

Published in India by: Hay House Publishers India, Muskaan Complex, Plot No. 3, B-2, Vasant Kunj, New Delhi 110 070
Phone: 91-11-4176-1620 • *Fax:* 91-11-4176-1630
www.hayhouse.co.in

Access New Knowledge.
Anytime. Anywhere.

Learn and evolve at your own pace
with the world's leading experts.

www.hayhouseU.com

Listen. Learn. Transform.

Listen to the audio version of this book for FREE!

Gain access to endless wisdom, inspiration, and encouragement from world-renowned authors and teachers—guiding and uplifting you as you go about your day. With the *Hay House Unlimited* Audio app, you can learn and grow in a way that fits your lifestyle . . . and your daily schedule.

With your membership, you can:

- Let go of old patterns, step into your purpose, live a more balanced life, and feel excited again.
- Explore thousands of audiobooks, meditations, immersive learning programs, podcasts, and more.
- Access exclusive audios you won't find anywhere else.
- Experience completely unlimited listening. No credits. No limits. No kidding.

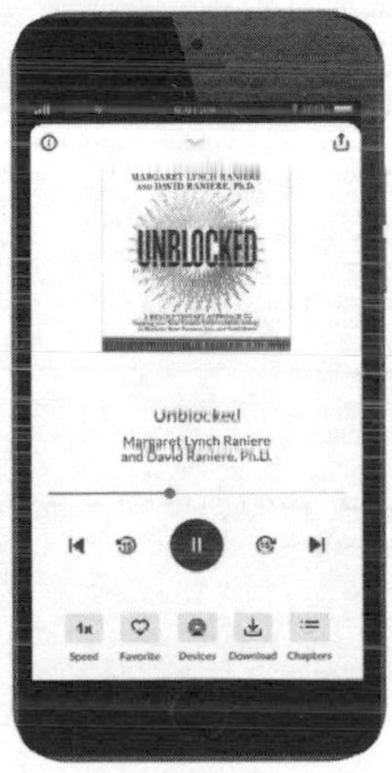

Try for FREE!

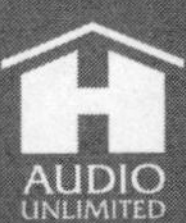

Visit hayhouse.com/listen-free to start your free trial and get one step closer to living your best life.

Free e-newsletters from Hay House, the Ultimate Resource for Inspiration

Be the first to know about Hay House's free downloads, special offers, giveaways, contests, and more!

Get exclusive excerpts from our latest releases and videos from ***Hay House Present Moments.***

Our ***Digital Products Newsletter*** is the perfect way to stay up-to-date on our latest discounted eBooks, featured mobile apps, and Live Online and On Demand events.

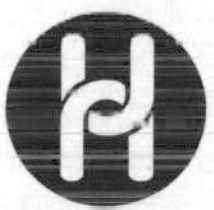

Learn with real benefits! ***HayHouseU.com*** is your source for the most innovative online courses from the world's leading personal growth experts. Be the first to know about new online courses and to receive exclusive discounts.

Enjoy uplifting personal stories, how-to articles, and healing advice, along with videos and empowering quotes, within ***Heal Your Life***.

Sign Up Now!

Get inspired, educate yourself, get a complimentary gift, and share the wisdom!

Visit www.hayhouse.com/newsletters to sign up today!

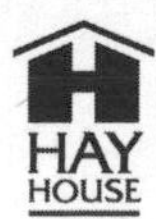

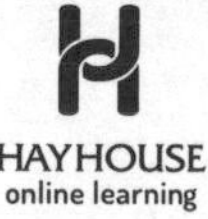